THE 4-WEEK
BODY BLITZ

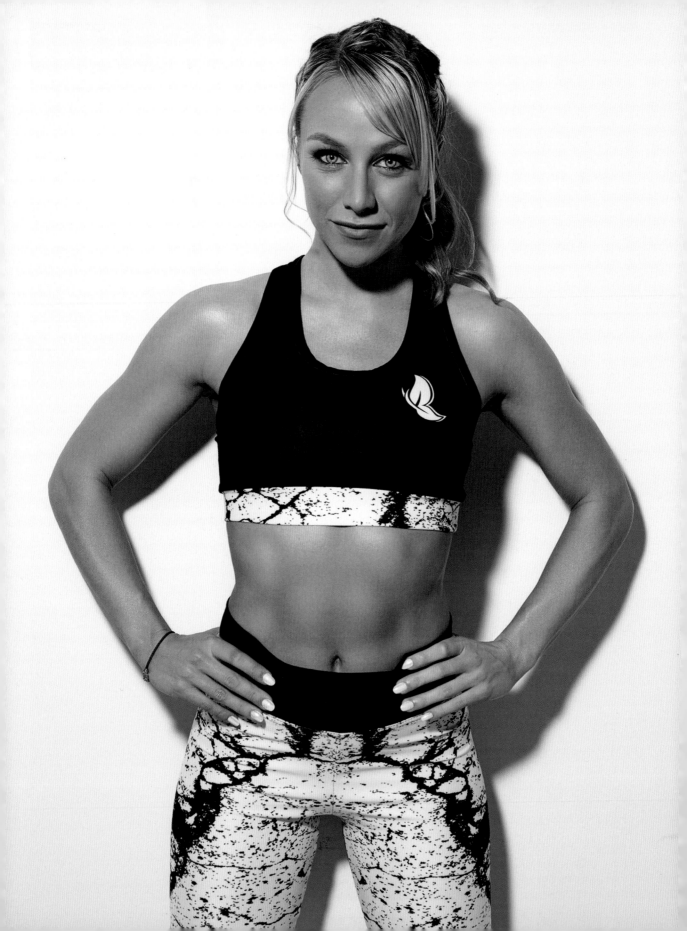

THE 4-WEEK BODY BLITZ

CHLOE MADELEY

Transform your body shape with my
complete diet and exercise plan

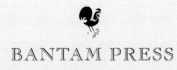

BANTAM PRESS

LONDON · NEW YORK · TORONTO · SYDNEY · AUCKLAND

TRANSWORLD PUBLISHERS
61–63 Uxbridge Road, London W5 5SA
www.penguin.co.uk

Transworld is part of the Penguin Random House group of companies
whose addresses can be found at global.penguinrandomhouse.com

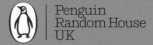
Penguin
Random House
UK

First published in Great Britain in 2017 by Bantam Press
an imprint of Transworld Publishers

Copyright © Chloe Madeley 2017

Chloe Madeley has asserted her right under the C
Designs and Patents Act 1988 to be identified as th

A CIP catalogue record for this book is available fr

ISBN 9780593079522

Project editor: Jo Roberts-Miller
Design: Smith & Gilmour
Cover and exercise photography by Sam Riley
Food photography by Smith & Gilmour

Typeset in Museo Slab 9.75/14pt by Smith & Gilmour
Printed and bound in Italy by Printer Trento S.r.l.

The health and fitness information in this book has been compiled by way
of general guidance in relation to the specific subjects addressed. It is not
intended as a substitute for medical advice. Please consult your GP or
healthcare professional before performing the exercises described in this
book, particularly if you are pregnant, elderly or have chronic or recurring
medical conditions. Do not attempt any of the exercises while under the
influence of alcohol or drugs. Discontinue any exercise that causes you
pain or severe discomfort and consult a medical expert. So far as the author
is aware the information given is correct and up to date at the time of
publication. The author and publishers disclaim, as far as the law allows,
any liability arising directly or indirectly from the use, or misuse, of the
information contained in this book.

Penguin Random House is committed to a sustainable
future for our business, our readers and our planet. This book
is made from Forest Stewardship Council® certified paper.

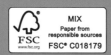
MIX
Paper from
responsible sources
FSC
www.fsc.org   FSC® C018179

1 3 5 7 9 10 8 6 4 2

CONTENTS

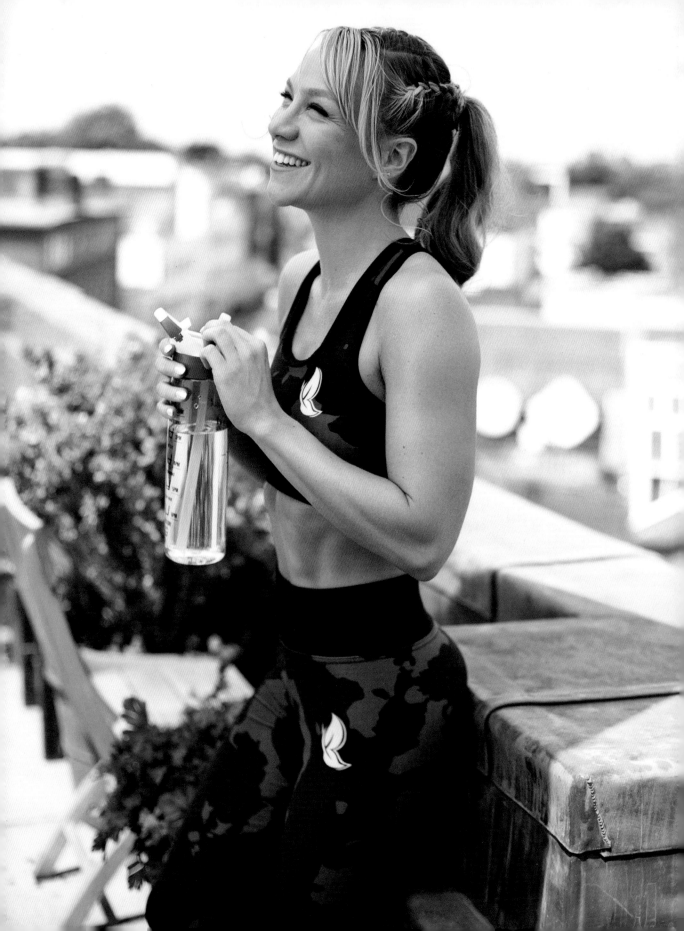

INTRODUCTION

A WORD FROM CHLOE

Hi, I'm Chloe Madeley, and welcome to *The 4-Week Body Blitz*.

Let me begin by telling you a bit about myself...

I started training properly and learning about nutrition in January 2013. I had just met my then boyfriend, who, luckily for me, was a personal trainer. I was a curvy size 10–12 and body confident, but my boyfriend asked if I'd like to be his aesthetic guinea pig to help him get some more female clients. I explained to him that I liked my body the way it was, and there was no changing it anyway – before a holiday I'd run daily and cut carbs for weeks on end, but my shape *never* changed. I was built the way I was built, period. He laughed and asked me what I was trying to achieve in these pre-holiday weeks...

Abs, I replied, before adding that abs were obviously genetic and I simply didn't have those genes.

He bet me he could change my body in 4 weeks, and I took the bet...

On day 1, he put an Olympic bar on my back and taught me how to squat.

That was it. I was hooked.

By week 2, I was crying like a baby because I wanted my old comfort foods back – wine, bread, cheese and chocolate.

By week 3, I was fully in the groove and I noticed my body finally starting to change.

By week 4, I had booked my place on a Personal Training course.

In June of that year, I started my blog FitnessFondue.com – I wanted to tell women what weight lifting felt like and what it was doing to my body. I wanted to explain how important nutrition is when it comes to changing your body.

Today, I have a big, beautiful fitness following, two best-selling training apps, a best-selling nutrition iBook, a supplement range and a gymwear line...

But *The 4-Week Body Blitz* is going to show you what I do best...

WHAT IS
THE 4-WEEK
BODY BLITZ?

Every health and fitness professional has a different approach to what they do.

There are the yogis who advocate a lifestyle change, daily meditation and cleansing superfood smoothies.

There are the body builders who lift heavy weights, manipulate hormone levels and pound protein shakes to get as big as humanly possible.

There are the cardio bunnies who challenge themselves with yearly marathons, triathlons and mountain hikes.

There are the gym socialites who take Spin, Bodypump and Metafit classes like they're going out of fashion.

And then there are the fitness models and coaches who specialise in time-sensitive body transformations.

This is what I do. This is what I *love*.

Body transformations would ideally take place over a 12–20-week time scale, and come off the back of months of effort to build as much muscle as humanly possible.

And it's not just fitness models who have to get in shape quickly for shoots and competitions. This short-term panic is *actually* very common amongst our clients and audience.

Whether it's the January fitness surge, the summer body quest or the Christmas party season, transformation time scales can often be staggeringly short.

Oh my God, I have a holiday next month!
How the hell am I going to fit into my wedding dress?!
If my ex is going to that party, I want to look amazing.

The 4-Week Body Blitz is an instructive guide designed to show you how to get into shape in the shortest time frame possible.

First, I'll explain how I'm going to help you alter what you eat and why; then comes my day-by-day stretching and exercise plan that shows you *exactly* what you need to do each day.

Don't worry, you're not going to have to do anything extreme – you will eat, you will train, and you will have rest days.

However, you must understand that with only 4 short weeks, there is absolutely no room for error.

We have 4 weeks to get you *the best results possible*.

And this means giving 110% to both your diet and training – *every single day.*

There is no time to mess around and no time to fall off the wagon.

There are 4 weeks to get the
job done, so let's get it done!

UNDERSTANDING THE RULES OF *THE 4-WEEK BODY BLITZ*

Before you start your new regime, I want to explain *why* the rules of *The 4-Week Body Blitz* are what they are.

I firmly believe that if you *understand* the process, you are much more likely to become invested in it and even excited by it.

UNDERSTANDING
YOUR NEW DIET

CLEAN EATING

Firstly, single ingredient foods (for example, eggs, oats, fruit, nuts, vegetables, chicken and fish) are a lot less calorie dense and more nutrient rich than processed foods, so you can actually eat a lot *more* than you might think in order to get fit and healthy.

For instance:
1 large chicken breast has ½ the calories of 2 small pork sausages, with none of the carbohydrates and roughly $1/14$th of the fat.
1 portion of berries has less than ½ the calories of 1 packet of sweets and none of the refined sugar.

Secondly, your body is able to *use* all the nutrients from unadulterated single ingredient foods, instead of storing wasted calories away as fat. Your body has no use for the excess sugars found in sweets and refined carbohydrates, or for the trans-fats found in most junk foods, so it has no choice other than to store them away, eventually forming adipose tissue, otherwise known as fat.

Lastly, you will be healthy from the inside out. Clean foods are rich in micronutrients (vitamins and minerals), which, surprisingly, tend to be missing from a bowl of French fries or a doughnut. Although your body may struggle without junk food for the first week or so, by week 3 you will feel great – I promise.

UNDERSTANDING TRAINING

Much like your new diet, I believe that if you *understand* what the specific exercises are doing to your body, you are much more likely to train hard and stay motivated.

There are 2 different types of training and they will change your body in 2 different ways:

1. CARDIOVASCULAR TRAINING – FAT BURNING

There are 3 different kinds of cardiovascular training:

›› *LISS (Low Intensity Steady State Cardio)*
An incline walk, a steady jog – anything that gets you puffing and sweating while being able to maintain your pace for long periods of time (typically 40–60 minutes).

›› *MISS (Moderate Intensity Steady State Cardio)*
An incline jog, a gentle run – anything that challenges you but that you can maintain for a period of time (typically 30–40 minutes).

›› *HIIT (High Intensity Interval Training)*
Interval sprints, burpees, mountain climbers, box jumps, fast-paced skipping – anything that you can give 100% effort to for no longer than a minute. You recover for the following minute and then repeat.

If you enjoy walking, cycling or horse riding, for example, please feel free to continue with them while also giving this blitz 100%!

2. RESISTANCE TRAINING – MUSCLE BUILDING

There are 2 different types of resistance training:

>> *Body Weight / Gravity*

Sit ups, squat jumps, push ups – using your body weight / gravity to challenge and fatigue your muscle.

>> *Weighted*

Dumbbells, barbells, kettlebells, medicine balls, machines – using external objects to challenge and fatigue your muscle.

This book uses circuit training to get both your (HIIT) cardio and resistance training done in one fell swoop. (Feel free to continue any classes / outdoor activities, like running or cycling, alongside this plan.)

It is designed to change your body regardless of what equipment you have available to you.

>> You do not need gym membership
>> You do not need a cardio machine
>> You do not need weights
>> You can do every exercise outdoors or in your living room.

However, if you *do* have equipment at home, then please feel free to use it. Whether you have a treadmill, a kettlebell, a medicine ball, *whatever*, if you can incorporate it into the exercises listed further on, then absolutely do.

If you have the energy to
carry on with your gym class
it will only help your results.

The 4-Week Body Blitz initially requires you to train for 5 days a week, eventually working your way up to 6 days. Please note that those of you who are just starting out and have low fitness levels can take the week 1 circuits nice and slow – *but you must complete them fully.*

Alternatively, for 2–3 weeks leading up to starting this plan, you might want to try LISS (Low Intensity Steady State) cardio (e.g. an incline walk, a steady jog – anything that gets you puffing and sweating) for 5–6 days each week for 40–60 minutes each day. HIIT cardio is hard and resistance training is hard, so building up some mental and physical tolerance before throwing yourself into circuit training might be a good plan of action.

For those of you who are already pretty fit, though, you have no excuse whatsoever. Go straight into week 1 giving 100% and absolutely *no less.* Keep that momentum up until your very last workout. No excuses. Period.

DOMS (DELAYED ONSET MUSCLE SORENESS)

You will probably find, even if you are used to training hard, that you develop DOMS in the first few days of starting this plan. DOMS happens when we switch up our training or start a new exercise routine, and it is a very GOOD sign. It means your muscle tissue has torn and is on the mend, which means training is working, your metabolic rate is increasing and you are on your way to that 'toned' defined look. Do NOT miss a training day because you are sore. Instead, stretch throughout the day, hydrate well, make sure your protein intake is high and get a good night's sleep. See DOMS as a pat on the back for training hard and keep going!

You may struggle to keep going with an exercise at a dynamic level for the full minute. If this happens, slow the movement down but don't stop. You must make sure you complete the entire minute, even if you need to switch to a more gentle movement.

YOU'VE GOT THIS!

The last thing I want to talk about is the mental, emotional and motivational 'journey' you are about to take.

The word 'journey' is cheesy and clichéd but it's also the best way to describe what the next 4 weeks are going to feel like for you.

The fact of the matter is, changing any habit is exciting at first, but it quickly becomes a challenge – and getting through that challenge is a mental battle.

There will be days when you genuinely don't think this is a good idea any more. There will be days when you're tired and you either *don't* want to train or you *do* want to eat cake – most likely simultaneously.

But you must keep going and stick with it.

Remember, habits don't start as habits, they start as daily efforts.
Remember *why* you started to make these daily efforts.
Visualise the results you want from these daily efforts.
Remember that they *will* eventually become habits.

Nobody becomes an Olympian overnight.
Nobody writes a best-selling novel in the first draft.
Nobody has ever achieved anything by giving up when it gets hard.

Junk food isn't going anywhere.
It was there last month and it will still be there next month.

I love chocolate. I love cake. I love pizza. I love pasta. I love wine.
I love cheese. I love lying very still for obscenely long periods of time.
So, if I can do this, anyone can.

Dig deep, find your inner warrior and fight for what you want!

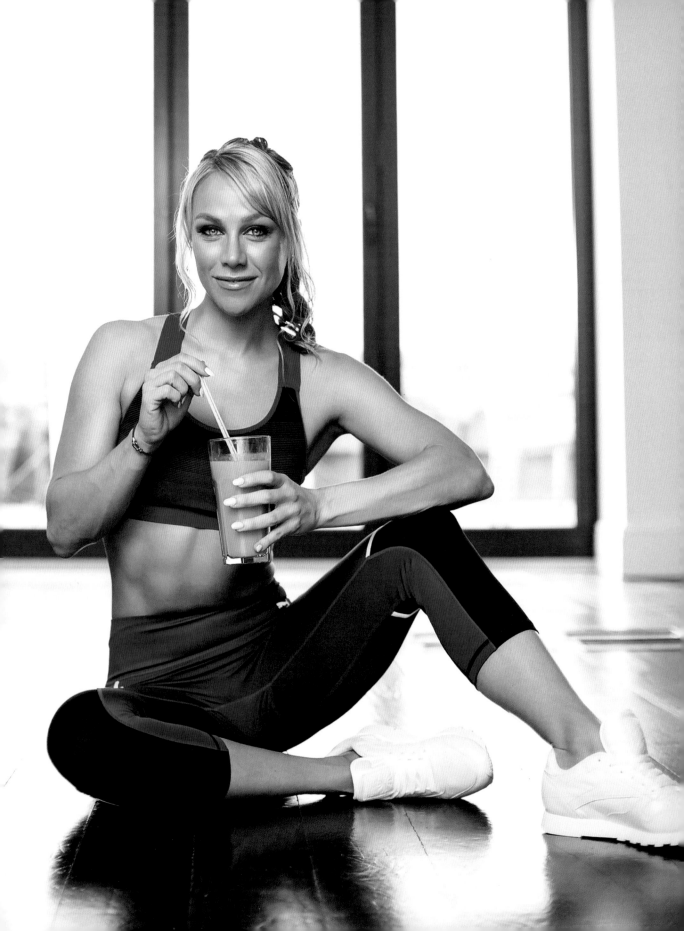

YOUR
NEW DIET

This book includes a meal plan for you to follow over the course of the next 4 weeks. It will determine your daily calorie intake, daily macro intake and weekly macro manipulation (otherwise known as carb cycling – this is all explained in the following pages!).

Your daily food intake is going to be as follows:

Breakfast

Snack (a.m.)

Lunch

Snack (p.m.)

Dinner

MACRONUTRIENTS

Our bodies need calories in order to survive. These calories should be made up of the 3 macronutrients:

1 Proteins

2 Fats

3 Carbohydrates

The right calorie count will ensure results.
And a good macro balance will ensure optimum
physical health and function.

I have structured your diet to ensure it is low calorie and has a balance of all 3 macronutrients, but you will need to follow the rules so you know **when** to eat each macro and **how much** of each macro to eat. This is because both the timing and quantity of food will ensure you get the best results possible over the course of the next 4 weeks.

Those of you who already know about calories and macros will know that there are ways to include daily treats into this type of diet while still achieving results but let me be absolutely clear now – this is **not** the case with *The 4-Week Body Blitz.*

Why?

We only have 4 weeks.

We will not be including cheats, such
as doughnuts and pizza.

Period.

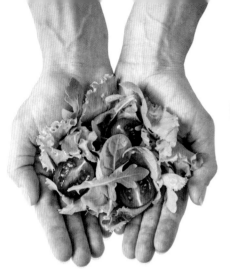 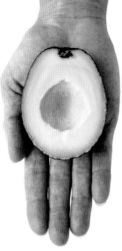 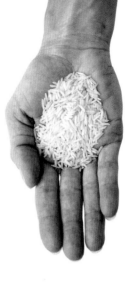 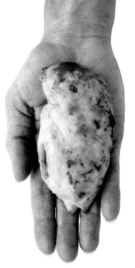

1 PORTION
Non-starchy veg
2 loosely cupped hands

1 PORTION
Fat
1 palm size

1 PORTION
Carb
1 palm size

1 PORTION
Protein
1 outstretched hand

PORTION CONTROL

Daily snacks and full plates of food are frequent on this diet but the meal sizes and snack quantities must be strictly adhered to – they have been calculated carefully to comprise your weekly calorie intake. Having an extra handful of nuts or a second lunch is going to add up to hundreds of calories or more – and that's absolutely NOT going to get you the results you want.

I have kept it simple for you, using hand sizes and spoon sizes so you don't have to weigh anything out. But *you must follow all measurements to the letter!*

A small handful of nuts will be 100 or so calories, while a large handful could be as much as 400. If you consistently give yourself more than you should, the calories will add up and you can say goodbye to your body transformation and hello to a plateau, or even a gain.

≫ Calorie control is essential to aesthetic results.

≫ Remember, this is just a short-term plan, but you need to stick to it!

BUILD YOUR OWN MEALS
AND SNACKS

Every day you need to make sure you have breakfast, lunch, dinner and two snacks – one in the morning and one in the afternoon. This will keep you full and will ensure that you are hitting the right calorie count.

You can use the recipes at the back of the book or you can build your own nutritious meals and snacks from scratch (see page 31). (This will be particularly useful for those of you who have special dietary requirements – vegetarians, gluten or lactose intolerant etc.)

The recipes themselves are simple and straightforward because I know time can be short, and each one has been written specifically for the plan, so you know that if you use them, you *will* see results.

When it comes to building your own meals, I'd like you to follow the hands and fists method of measuring to ensure you don't overeat (see photos opposite and explanation on page 28). Remember – if you consistently over-estimate your handfuls, you can say goodbye to your body transformation.

Everybody is different but I tend to find a meal I like (Chicken Sausage and Broccoli Mash on page 171, for example) and eat it for most meals until I'm bored. Obviously, you don't have to do this but it does make life easier and guarantee enjoyable meal times!

CARB CYCLING

FAT   CARB   FAT   CARB

HIGH FAT & LOW CARB OR HIGH CARB & LOW FAT?

You will notice that over the course of the 4 weeks, there are changes to your weekly carbohydrate intake...

Welcome to the wonderful world of carb cycling!

WHAT IS CARB CYCLING?

Carb cycling is a great dietary tool used by those who train regularly with the goal to simultaneously shed fat and maintain muscle mass. It can either mean timing your starchy carbohydrate intake around training (pre and post), or going a period of days (usually between 3–7) on a low/no carbohydrate diet, before then 'refeeding' on a selected high carb day.

WHY DO IT?

Carb cycling works particularly well when it comes to shedding fat, feeding muscle and boosting hormone and metabolic levels.

HOW DOES IT WORK?

Your body converts carbohydrates into glucose, which it then burns for immediate energy. Excess glucose is stored in your liver and muscles as glycogen, which your body will turn to later when it needs an energy boost. Excess glycogen will eventually be released back into the body and stored as adipose tissue (body fat).

However, if your body has depleted both its glucose and glycogen stores, it is then going to become much more efficient at burning fat for energy. By going several days on a low / no carbohydrate diet, your body will start using its fat stores for energy.

However, if you train hard while on a low carb intake, it's only a matter of time before your body starts to struggle. Why? Because, as I said, glycogen is stored in your liver and muscles and if your glycogen stores are depleted, your muscles will feel flat and weak. Training is hard as it is, but if your muscles are weak, it is torturous.

As well as contributing to muscular weakness and depletion, low calorie and low carbohydrate diets will also eventually floor your hormone levels, including a hormone called leptin, which controls your metabolism. Once your leptin levels are down, your metabolic rate is going to come to a screeching halt, and you can say goodbye to your ongoing body transformation.

By refeeding on a selected day with a surplus of carbohydrates, your muscles will fill, your hormone levels and metabolic rate will skyrocket, and you can continue to train hard and burn fat effectively over the next few days.

But don't panic – on each day of the plan I'll show you whether you are on a high carb or high fat day. I've worked it all out so that you don't have to!

YOUR CARB CYCLE

WEEK 1

(every 4th day)
Starchy carb meals and snacks will be restricted to and reserved for – **Thursday**

MONDAY

FAT · CARB

TUESDAY

FAT CARB

WEDNESDAY

FAT CARB

THURSDAY

CARB FAT

FRIDAY

FAT CARB

SATURDAY

FAT CARB

SUNDAY

FAT CARB

WEEK 2

(every 4th day)
Starchy carb meals and snacks will be restricted to and reserved for – **Monday and Friday**

MONDAY

CARB FAT

TUESDAY

FAT CARB

WEDNESDAY

FAT CARB

THURSDAY

FAT CARB

FRIDAY

CARB FAT

SATURDAY

FAT CARB

SUNDAY

FAT CARB

WEEK 3

(every 5th day)
Starchy carb meals and snacks will be restricted
to and reserved for – **Wednesday**

MONDAY

FAT CARB

TUESDAY

FAT CARB

WEDNESDAY

CARB FAT

THURSDAY

FAT CARB

FRIDAY

FAT CARB

SATURDAY

FAT CARB

SUNDAY

FAT CARB

WEEK 4

(every 5th day)
Starchy carb meals and snacks will be restricted
to and reserved for – **Monday and Saturday**

MONDAY

CARB FAT

TUESDAY

FAT CARB

WEDNESDAY

FAT CARB

THURSDAY

FAT CARB

FRIDAY

FAT CARB

SATURDAY

CARB FAT

SUNDAY

FAT CARB

FAT   **CARB**

HIGH FAT &
LOW CARB DAYS

**EVERY MEAL
(Breakfast + Lunch
+ Dinner + Snacks)**
1 portion protein + 1 portion
non-starchy vegetables
+ 1 portion fats

1 portion of PROTEIN =
1 outstretched hand (eg 1 large
chicken breast / 1 large fish fillet /
1 small steak / ½ small pack
lean mince etc)

**1 portion of NON-STARCHY
VEGETABLES =** 2 loosely cupped
hands (leaves, broccoli, cauliflower,
onions, tomatoes, cucumber,
mushrooms, peppers etc)

1 portion of FATS =
1 palm size
(eg 2 small eggs /
½ small avocado /
1 small handful nuts etc)

See page 22 for portion sizes

CARB   **FAT**

HIGH CARB &
LOW FAT DAYS

**EVERY MEAL
(Breakfast + Lunch
+ Dinner + Snacks)**
1 portion protein + 1 portion
non-starchy vegetables
+ 1 portion starchy carbs / fruit

1 portion of PROTEIN =
1 outstretched hand (eg 1 large
chicken breast / 1 large fish fillet /
1 small steak / ½ small pack
lean mince etc)

**1 portion of NON-STARCHY
VEGETABLES =** 2 loosely cupped
hands (leaves, broccoli, cauliflower,
onions, tomatoes, cucumber,
mushrooms, peppers etc)

**1 portion of STARCHY CARBS /
FRUIT =** 1 palm size
(eg 1 handful rice /
1 handful oats / 1 small potato /
1 small portion fruit etc)

See page 22 for portion sizes

MEN & *THE 4-WEEK BODY BLITZ*

All the quantities given here are for
an average woman. Men will need
to increase their food intake by ½.

In other words,
every **HIGH FAT LOW CARB** day
men should be eating:
1½ portions protein
+ 1½ portions non-starchy vegetables
+ 1½ portions fats
For every meal and snack

And every **HIGH CARB LOW FAT** day
they should be eating
1½ portions protein
+ 1½ portions non-starchy vegetables
+ 1½ portions starchy carbs / fruit
For every meal and snack

See page 22 for portion sizes

YOUR FOOD BIBLE

I have listed all the foods
you will be allowed to eat over
the course of the next 4 weeks
in the table opposite.

I have separated these foods
into 3 sections:

1 Proteins (dominant macro)

2 Fats (secondary macro)

3 Carbohydrates (cycled macro)

You will notice that there are plenty of protein, fat and carb food
options that are not included in the list opposite. It may seem strict,
but foods such as pork bacon, pork sausages, cheeses, pastas, breads
etc are going to be off limits for a few weeks.

The truth is that you can eat *any* food and still get in shape. However,
the foods I have included in the plan will provide the right amount
of calories *and* are of better nutritional value.

There is a lot of debate as to whether a clean diet or a calorie-controlled
diet is better. *The 4-Week Body Blitz* involves both because I want you
to lose weight *and* become 100% healthy from the inside out. In order
to succeed at this, you need to be well fed *and* always feel full.

FOODS PERMITTED ON *THE 4-WEEK BODY BLITZ*

PROTEINS	FATS	CARBOHYDRATES
Egg Whites	Whole Eggs	**EVERYDAY CARBS**
0% Fat Greek Yoghurt	Avocados	All Non-Starchy Vegetables (leaves / greens / onions / broccoli / cauliflower / cucumber / mushrooms / artichokes / asparagus / bamboo shoots / bean sprouts / celery / sprouts / cabbage / leeks / okra / peppers / radishes / tomato)
All Fish (salmon / tuna / cod / haddock)	All Nuts / Seeds	
	All Clean Nut Butters (no added oils / sugars)	
Chicken (breast / sausage)	Oils (olive / sesame / coconut)	
Turkey (breast / bacon /mince)	Oily / Fatty Fish (salmon etc)	**HIGH CARB DAYS ONLY**
Lean Beef Mince (5%)	Dark Chocolate (90%)	All Starchy Vegetables (potatoes / parsnips / plantain / pumpkin / corn / peas / beans / lentils)
Lean Steak Cuts (fillet /medallions)	Fatty Steak Cuts (sirloin)	
Whey Protein Powder	Fatty Beef Mince (15%)	All Fruit (berries and bananas are best)
Soy Protein (tofu etc – in moderation)	Full Fat Greek Yoghurt	All Rice
All Mycoprotein (Quorn pieces / mince)	Butter	Puffed Rice Cereals (clean – no added sugars)
		Rice Cakes (clean – no added sugars)
		Popcorn (clean – no added sugars)
		Oats

ADDITIONS AND SEASONING

You can use the ingredients below to enhance the flavour of the dishes you cook. But only use the quantities given here – otherwise the calories will creep up.

>> ½ x 400g tin chopped tomatoes

>> 1 level tbsp 0% fat Greek yoghurt

>> 1 tbsp lemon / lime juice

>> 1 tbsp soy sauce

>> 1 level tbsp reduced sugar ketchup

>> 1 level tsp agave / stevia

>> 1 tbsp vinegar

>> 1 stock cube

>> 1 tsp mustard

>> 1 tbsp gravy granules

>> 1 tsp hot sauce (such as Tabasco)

>> Salt / pepper / garlic / ginger / chilli / herbs / spices

DRINKS

During *The 4-Week Body Blitz*, you'll need to be careful about what you drink, as well as what you eat, otherwise you'll find that your calorie intake will creep up.

So you're going to need to stick to the following:

>> Unsweetened almond milk / Unsweetened coconut milk / Unsweetened cashew milk / Skimmed milk (in moderation)

>> Tea

>> Coffee

>> Water

>> Diet drinks (in moderation)

WATER

It's not all about food. Your water intake is going to play a vital role in changing your body.

The human body is made up of around 60% water, your muscles are around 80% water, and your lungs carry even more than that. So imagine how good you will feel if you feed your body a constant flow of fresh water, pushing nutrients around your body efficiently and hydrating your muscles continuously. Then imagine how that is going to end up *looking* on you externally.

I recommend that you try to drink **4 litres of water a day** – that means a couple of large cups of tea or coffee and 1 litre with every meal (breakfast, lunch and dinner). My number one piece of advice is to buy yourself a 1-litre bottle and make sure 1 litre is already down you before you sit down to each meal. I find it is better to space out the consumption of each litre as much as possible.

SLEEP

The last factor you need to consider when it comes to changing your body is sleep.

Most of us struggle to make it through even a lazy day on only a few hours of sleep, so imagine how you're going to feel when you start throwing daily / weekly training into the equation. Your body needs rest as much as it needs movement. Sleep is when your body recovers, in terms of hormonal and muscular changes – both *critical* to your aesthetic results. If you notice that your body isn't changing but you have been sticking 100% to the diet and training plan, you can bet it's a lack of water or sleep that's holding you back.

You have to *try* for at least **8 hours of sleep a night**. If you really struggle to do this because of kids and / or work, just keep *trying* to achieve it. You might surprise yourself.

SUPPLEMENTS

No – you do not need supplements to change your body.
Yes – they can aid your training and recovery.

Pre-workouts (caffeine supplements) can be helpful if you feel sluggish in the mornings or after work. This can be in the form of good, old-fashioned caffeine, or as a supplement called a **Thermogenic**. However, as I said, a strong black coffee or large green tea will work just as well.

For those of you who dislike drinking water and struggle to give up sugary drinks, **BCAAs** (branch chain amino acids – aka proteins) are a great supplement that come in flavoured powder form which you dissolve in water. It can be quite hit and miss finding a flavour you like but, once you find one, it makes water consumption so much easier. BCAAs will feed your muscle throughout the day and during your workouts.

The diet plan allows for **Protein Powder**, but not *all* protein powders are suitable. Look for options that range between 90–120 kcals per 1 serving / scoop and that are high in protein but low in fats and carbs. This typically looks like 15–30g protein and 1–5g fats and / or carbs per serving. Look out for **'diet' whey, '100%' whey, 'isolate' whey and 'impact' whey** – these tend to be the right choices.

Fish Oils or **Omega Oils** are really going to help you in terms of your joint health, cardiovascular health and muscular recovery. I take one with every meal.

There is no scientific evidence that **Multivitamins** work, but if you are challenging your body in a new way with daily training, your immune system can take a hit. Since I started taking multivits, I haven't had a single cold.

SPECIAL DIETARY NEEDS

Vegetarians can substitute all animal protein sources with any complete protein source that is **not** a starch. In other words, rice and beans would not be permitted as an animal protein substitute but there are some complete protein sources you could use:

>> Mycoprotein (such as Quorn)
>> Soy protein (such as tofu)
>> Egg whites
>> 0% fat Greek yoghurt
>> Protein powders (whey, casein or pea)

Please be aware that vegetables are **not** *complete* protein sources (essential amino acids) and therefore do not count as protein replacements.

For those of you with gluten intolerances and other digestive problems, it is fine to replace one food option with another, so long as you have the following in your daily diet:

1 Complete protein source
2 Vegetable source
3 Fatty acid source (high fat days only)
4 Starchy carb source (high carb days only)

See page 31 for examples of each food group.

SNACK OPTIONS FOR WOMEN

Choose 2 of these snack options to have each day –
1 mid morning and 1 mid afternoon.

>> 1 small pot 0% fat Greek yoghurt (typically 170g)

>> 1 protein shake (1 scoop with water and / or ice)

>> 1 small packet cooked chicken (typically 100g)

>> 1 small packet cooked prawns (typically 150g)

>> 1 small packet beef jerky (typically 28g)

>> 2 squares 90% dark chocolate (typically 25g each)

>> 1 small bag kale crisps / kale chips (typically 15g)

LOW CARB DAYS ONLY

>> 1 small handful any nuts (typically 20g)

>> 1 level tbsp any clean nut butter

>> ½ avocado

>> 2 small boiled eggs

HIGH CARB DAYS ONLY

>> 2 rice cakes (no added sugar)

>> 1 sachet / 1 heaped tbsp oats

>> 1 small bag popcorn (no added oils / sugar – typically 17g)

>> 1 small piece fruit

♂

SNACK OPTIONS FOR MEN

Choose 2 of these snack options to have each day –
1 mid morning and 1 mid afternoon.

>> 1½ small pots 0% fat Greek yoghurt (typically 250g)

>> 1 protein shake (1½ scoops with water and / or ice)

>> 1½ small packets cooked chicken (typically 150g)

>> 1½ small packets cooked prawns (typically 225g)

>> 1½ small packets beef jerky (typically 42g)

>> 3 squares 90% dark chocolate (typically 25g each)

>> 2 small bags kale crisps / kale chips (typically 30g)

LOW CARB DAYS ONLY

>> 1½ small handfuls any nuts (typically 30g)

>> 1 heaped tbsp any clean nut butter

>> ¾ avocado

>> 3 small boiled eggs

HIGH CARB DAYS ONLY

>> 3 rice cakes (no added sugar)

>> 1½ sachets / 2 tbsp oats

>> 2 small bags popcorn (no added oils / sugar – typically 17g each)

>> 2 small pieces fruit

TO MAKE YOUR OWN POPCORN

Place a heavy-based pan over a medium heat and add a large handful of corn kernels. Cover with a tight-fitting lid and heat. The kernels will start to pop – leave over the heat until the popping sound dies out. Remove the pan from the heat and carefully remove the lid. Sprinkle the popcorn with a little salt while it's still warm.

TO MAKE YOUR OWN KALE CHIPS

Preheat the oven to 150°C. Wash 100g kale leaves (tough stalks removed) and dry thoroughly. Place in a bowl and tear any large leaves. Sprinkle with ras el hanout, or a similar spice, and some sea salt, and mix well. Line 2 baking trays with baking parchment and tip the kale onto the trays. Spread out into a single layer and bake for 18–22 minutes, or until crisp but still green. Leave to cool for a few minutes and then enjoy.

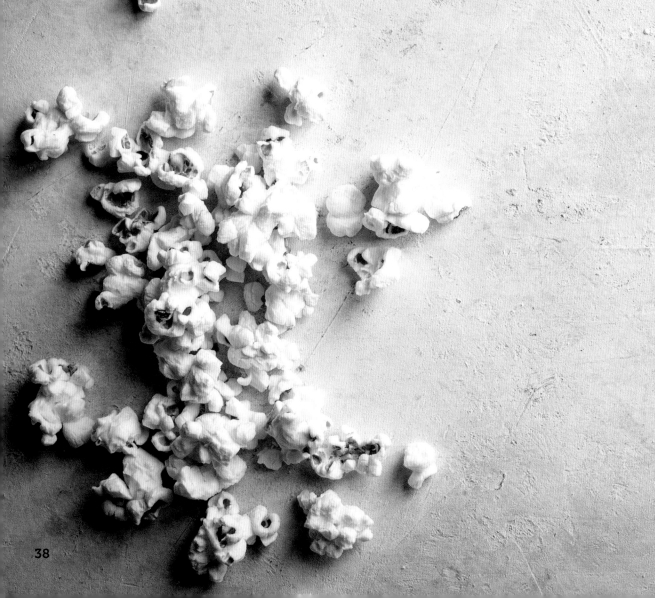

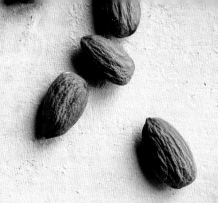

MAKING YOUR NEW DIET WORK WITH WORK

It goes without saying that you can't cook a lunch at work as easily as you can at home. But there are a couple of good ways to stay on track while at work:

>> Buy foods that you know fit into your food bible, portion size and carb cycle instructions. For example, on a low carb, high fat day you could have a chicken avocado salad or a sashimi platter. On a high carb, low fat day you could have a small sushi platter, or a side of sweet potato wedges with your salad. Take time to look at menus, think about the food options, don't rush, don't panic, and if you have to order something without the fries – DO.

>> Cook double, triple, even quadruple quantities of the recipes for your dinner (or over a lazy weekend), and then you have the next few days / nights sorted in terms of meal options. This is called meal prep, and I do it every few days without fail.

It can be really hard, particularly for those of you who have office jobs, to avoid all the naughty snacks that are available at work. It is a great idea to come prepared:

>> Bring your own snacks from home
>> Keep snacks in your fridge at work, or on your desk
>> Buy snacks when you buy your lunch – most supermarkets and shops carry all the options listed

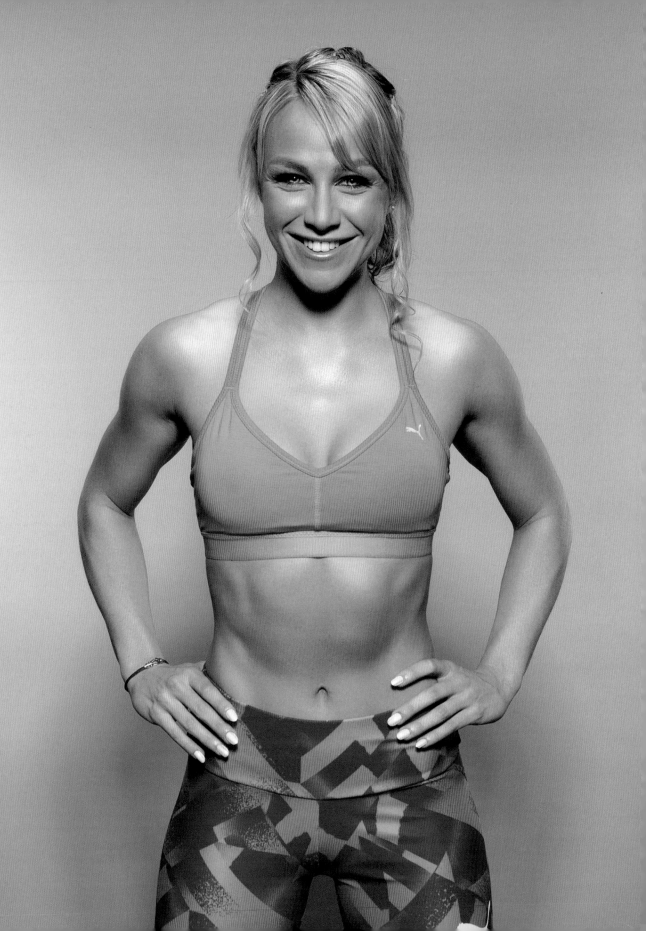

THE 4-WEEK BODY BLITZ

YOUR DAY-BY-DAY EXERCISE PLAN

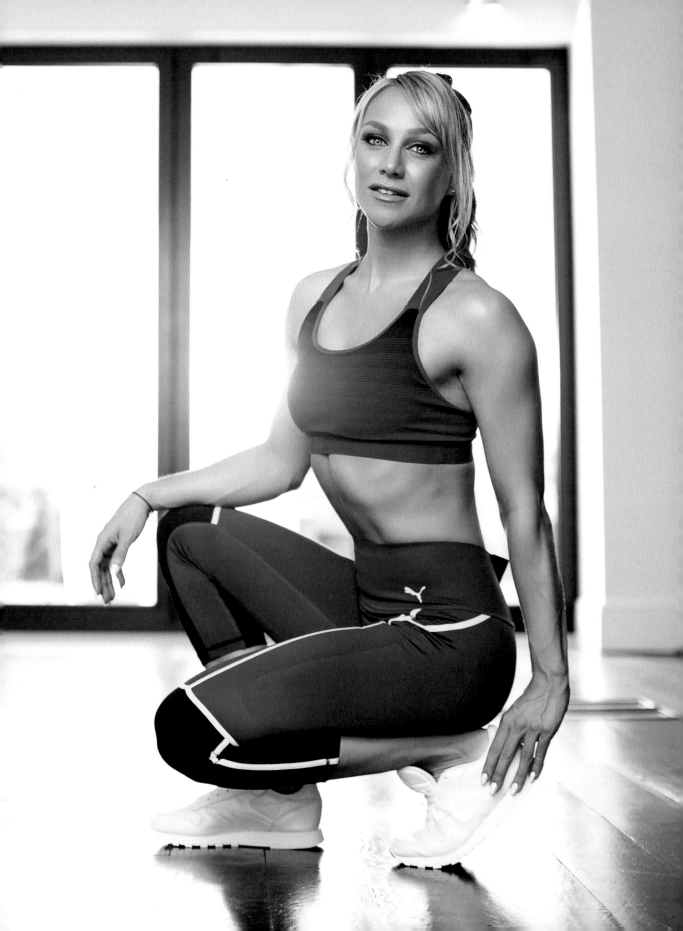

STRETCHING

You **must** warm up before and cool down after every training session.

Think of your body as a piece of chewing gum – if it's cold and you bend it, it will snap. If it's warm and you bend it, it will be supple and move.

Please note:
Warm up stretches are performed dynamically, meaning with a slow and gentle bouncy movement.

To make a stretch dynamic, hold the position and perform a gentle bounce as you do so, for 8–10 repetitions.

Cool down stretches are performed statically, meaning still.

To make a stretch static, hold the position still for 8–10 seconds.

Some of the stretches are for warming up only, most are for both warming up and cooling down. All the stretches are labelled so you know which are which.

SHOULDER STRETCH

WARM UP ONLY Stand up straight with your feet hip-width apart. Let your arms hang down by your sides. Place one hand across your body, rest it gently on the opposite side of your chest. In a slow, circular motion, lift your other arm out in front of you, then vertically up into the air. Let it gently continue the circle behind your body, and then complete the circle by letting it hang by your side where it started. Repeat this circular motion 8–10 times and then perform with the opposite arm.

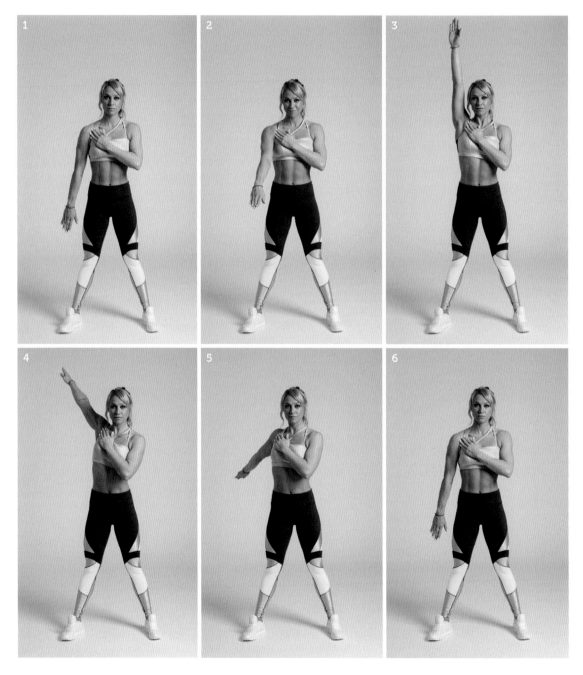

SHOULDER STRETCH

WARM UP & COOL DOWN

Stand up straight with your feet hip-width apart. Let your arms hang down by your sides. Lift one arm out in front of you. Reach your opposite hand across your body, under your armpit, and flatten your hand behind the extended arm's shoulder. Slowly and gently use your flattened hand to push against the back of the shoulder, extending the arm across your upper body, so it is horizontal across your chest. Repeat with the opposite arm.

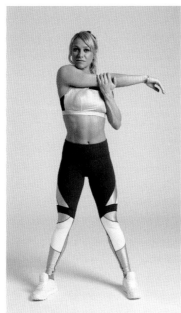 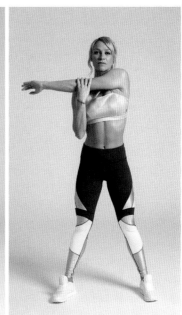

TRICEP STRETCH

WARM UP & COOL DOWN

Stand up straight with your feet hip-width apart. Lift one arm up into the air and then allow your forearm to hang down gently behind your head and neck. Using your opposite hand, gently grasp the back of your elbow / tricep area. Slowly push against this area so you feel a pull / stretch in your arm. Repeat with the opposite arm.

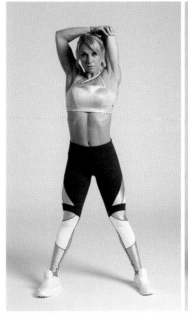 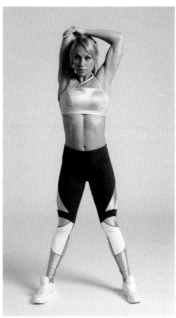

WRIST STRETCH

WARM UP ONLY Stand up straight with your feet hip-width apart. Extend both arms out to the sides (maintain a slight bend in your elbows). Slowly and gently roll your wrists outwards and inwards, in clockwise and anticlockwise movements respectively. Repeat this movement for 8–10 seconds.

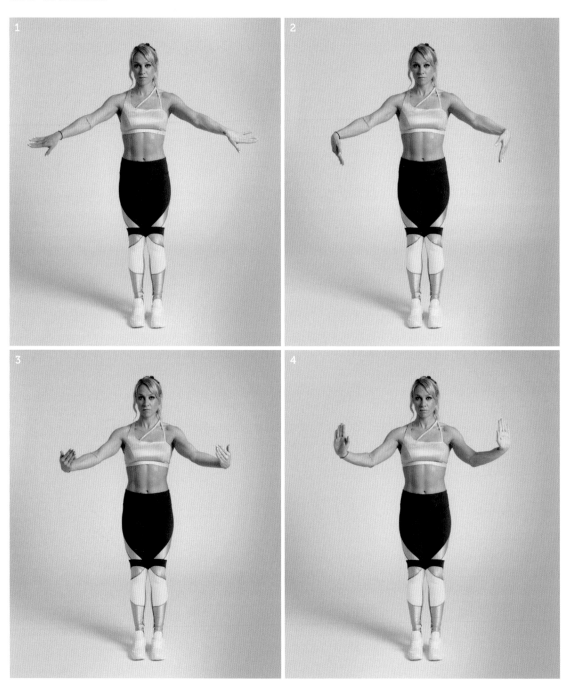

NECK STRETCH

WARM UP Stand up straight with your feet hip-width apart. Look straight ahead, then slowly and gently turn your head to one side, before coming back to centre. Then slowly and gently turn your head to the opposite side, before coming back to centre once again. Then look down, before coming back to centre, and finally look up, before coming back to centre again.

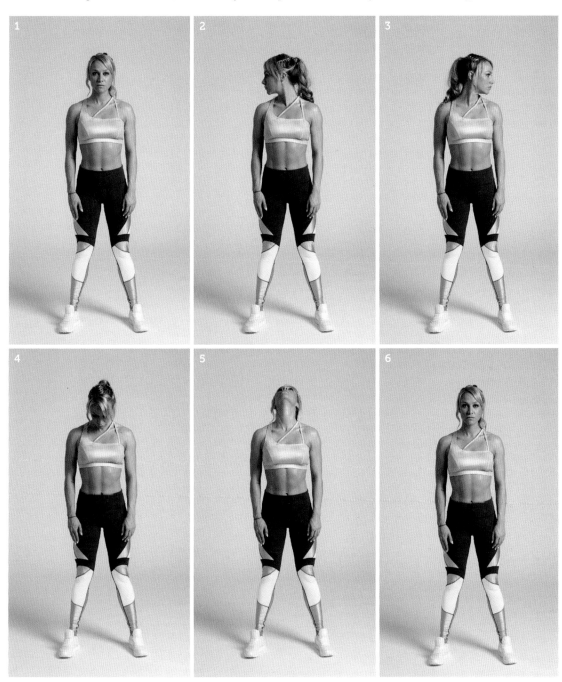

QUAD STRETCH

WARM UP & COOL DOWN
You may need to hold on
to something to keep your
balance while doing this.
Stand up straight with your
feet together. Bend one knee,
lifting one foot up behind
your body, and grasp the
foot with your hand. Slowly
and gently pull your foot
upwards, so you feel a pull /
stretch down the front of
your leg / quad. Repeat
this movement with your
opposite leg.

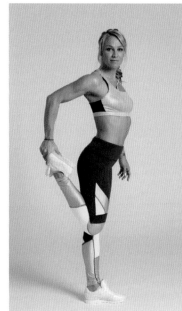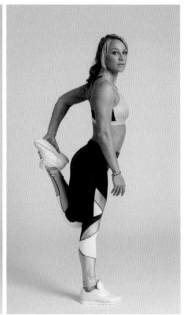

KNEE CIRCLES

WARM UP ONLY Stand with your feet together and bend down slightly so your hands fit
in between your knees. Gently circle the knees in a clockwise direction 8 times, before
repeating in the opposite direction.

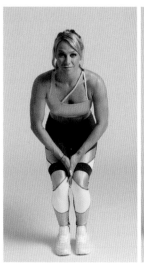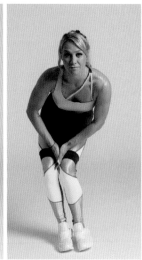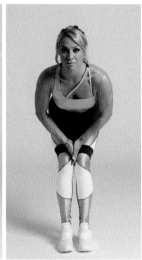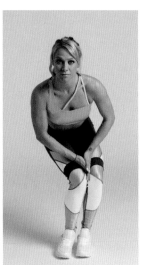

HAMSTRING STRETCH

WARM UP & COOL DOWN
Stand up straight with your feet together. Slowly and gently bend one knee (rest your hands on this knee to balance or, alternatively, place your hands on your hips). Slowly and gently stretch the opposite leg out in front of you, resting on the heel, toes pointing upwards. Keep your shoulders relaxed and feel the stretch in the back of your outstretched leg / hamstring. Repeat this movement with your opposite leg. Repeat with each leg 8–10 times to warm up. Hold each stretch for 8–10 seconds to cool down.

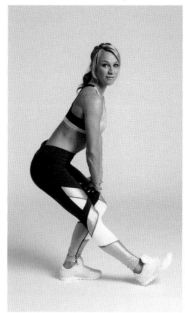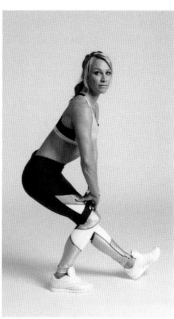

HIP OPENER

WARM UP & COOL DOWN Stand with your legs apart, toes facing outwards. Keeping your back straight / upright at all times, slowly and gently come down into a low squat. Rest your elbows on your knees for balance. Slowly and gently lean to the right, stretching your left hip out. Repeat on each side 8–10 times to warm up. Hold each stretch for 8–10 seconds to cool down.

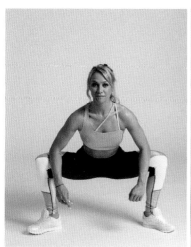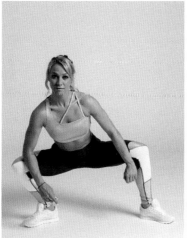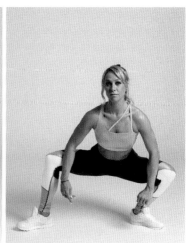

GLUTE STRETCH

WARM UP & COOL DOWN
Stand on your left leg and place your right ankle on top of your left thigh. Lower yourself down into a seated position – you will feel the stretch in the right side of your glute (buttocks). You can help the stretch by pressing gently on top of your right knee. Repeat with the opposite leg. If you have trouble keeping your balance, you can find something to hold on to.

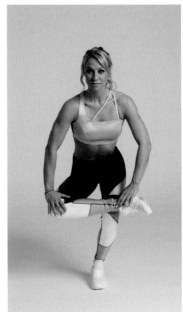
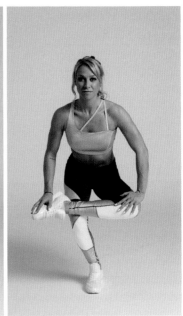

CALF STRETCH

WARM UP & COOL DOWN
Stand up straight with your feet together. Place your hands on your hips and lunge forward on one leg, as far as you can within your natural range. Keeping your back leg straight, try and push your back heel down to the ground – you should feel a stretch / pull in your calf muscle. Repeat with the opposite leg.

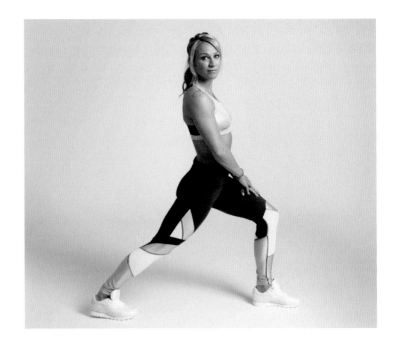

CHEST / BACK STRETCH

WARM UP ONLY Stand up straight with your feet hip-width apart. Raise your arms up to chest height and slowly and gently try to touch your elbows behind your back, within your natural range. Slowly and gently bring your arms back in front of your chest and cross your arms, almost like you are giving yourself a hug. Repeat this movement 8–10 times.

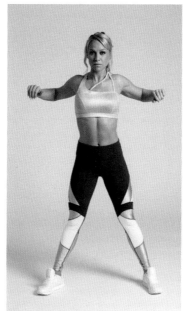 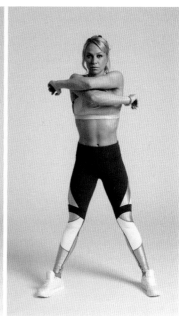

CHEST / BACK STRETCH

WARM UP & COOL DOWN Stand up straight with your feet hip-width apart. Let your arms hang loose at your sides before gently holding your hands behind your back. Slowly and gently extend your arms behind you, within your natural range, and try to pull your shoulders back and push your chest out.

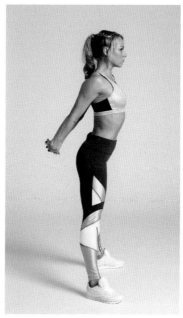 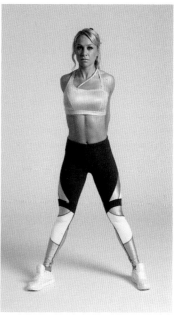

ANKLE ROLLS

WARM UP ONLY Using a simple circular motion, rotate each foot at the ankle for 10 circuits in each direction.

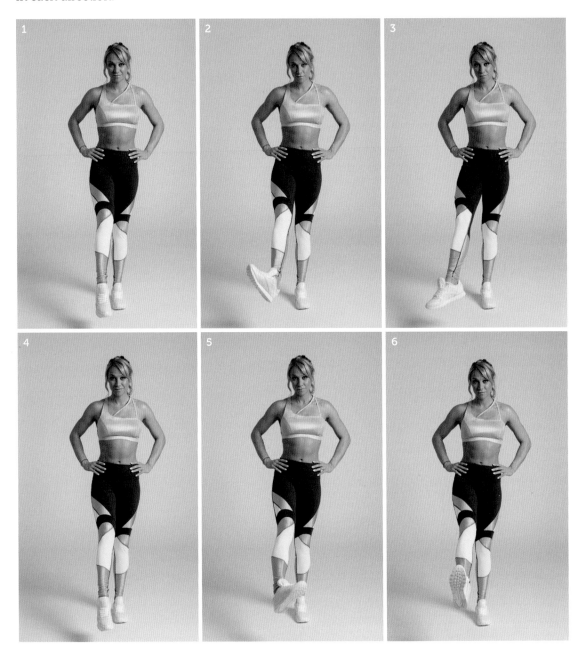

BACK STRETCH

WARM UP & COOL DOWN
Stand up straight with your
feet hip-width apart.
Crossing your arms in front
of you, let them wrap all the
way around your chest, like
you are giving yourself a
hug. With your hands flat
against the backs of your
shoulders, perform a gentle
pull – you should feel this
stretch in the centre of your
back. Slowly bend down,
creating a convex shape
with your spine.

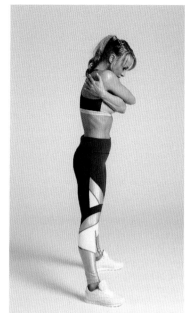
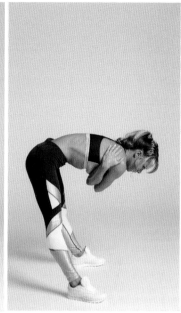

BICEP STRETCH

WARM UP & COOL DOWN
Stand up straight with your
feet hip-width apart. Raise
one arm out in front of you,
your fingertips pointing
upwards, your palm facing
forwards. Place your
opposite arm slightly above
the other, your fingertips
facing downwards, your
palm facing inwards. Slide
this hand over the other and
slowly and gently pull. You
will feel a stretch along the
inside of your arm. Repeat
with the opposite arm.

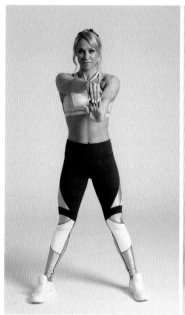
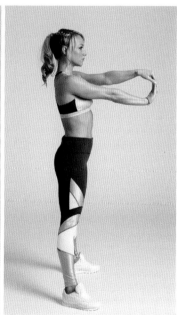

AB STRETCH

WARM UP & COOL DOWN Stand up straight with your feet hip-width apart. Raise your arms up above your head and lace your fingers together, palms facing the ceiling. Extend your upper body as much as you can within your range. You should feel a stretch up the front of your torso and also up the back of your spine. After holding this position for 8–10 seconds, keep your back straight and slowly and gently bend outwards to one side. You will feel a pull along the side of your torso. Repeat on the opposite side.

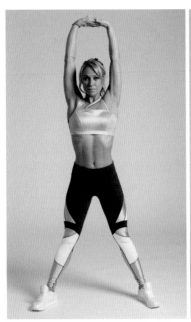 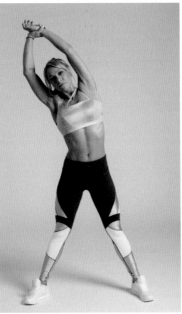 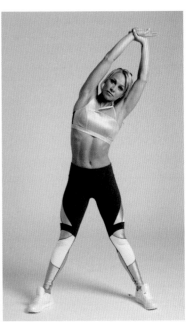

Listen to your favourite music as you warm up so you can start to 'catch the buzz' for training. As soon as that timer starts, attack your circuit like a boss – take charge and ENJOY YOURSELF!

TRAINING

You don't have to perform Monday's circuit on Monday – you could swap it for Thursday's, for example – but be sure you've done each of the 4 circuits during the week and make sure you perform the **exercises** within each circuit in the **order** specified – we're alternating cardiovascular with resistance training.

You can perform these workouts at any time of day – it really does not matter what time you train. However, I usually recommend getting your training done before breakfast (otherwise known as fasted) for 2 reasons:

Life is busy, it's unpredictable and it's not always easy to find time to train. Getting up early and getting your training done before you start your day means it's already done – the first box of the day is ticked. Nothing can get in the way of it and you'll have no opportunity to procrastinate.

After we train, our metabolism is revved up. Therefore, if you train before breakfast, your first meal of the day is already going straight to good use.

The theory goes that with no food for your body to burn for fuel, it's more likely to burn those stubborn fat stores for energy. The arguments for fasted training equating to greater fat burning are unproven, but they are propounded by many and are worth considering.

However, I must reiterate: it does *not* matter
if you can only train in your lunch break or in
the evenings. Burning 500 calories at 7am is just
as effective as burning 500 calories at 7pm.

Morning or night – just get it done.

WEEK 1
5 DAYS x 30 MINUTES

WEEK 2
5 DAYS x 35 MINUTES

WEEK 3
5 DAYS x 40 MINUTES

WEEK 4
6 DAYS x 40 MINUTES

WEEK

Welcome to *The 4-Week Body Blitz*.
Good luck and try to enjoy it!

**You'll see that every exercise has an illustration
and an explanation to show you how to do it.
You need to perform each circuit 6 times, bringing
the daily workout to a total of 30 minutes,
plus warm up and cool down time.**

Please note: You may struggle to keep going with
the exercise at a dynamic level for the full minute. If this
happens, slow the movement down but don't stop! You
must make sure you complete the entire minute of the
exercise, even if you need to switch to gentle movement.

WARM UP
(see pages 43–54)

EXERCISES 1–4
back to back and then rest for 1 minute
Total: 5 minutes

REPEAT
exercises 1–4 followed by a rest x 6 times
Total: 30 minutes

COOL DOWN
(see pages 43–54)

1 SQUAT JUMPS x 1 minute

Stand up straight with your feet hip-width apart. Extend your arms directly out in front of you and place one hand on top of the other – alternatively, place your hands on your hips. Keeping your back straight, lower yourself down into a deep squat by bending your knees. Instead of standing back up again from the squat, gently jump back into a standing position. The jump should be so gentle that you can maintain your form from the very start of the exercise to the next repetition. It should also be so gentle that you only come off the floor a little. Bear in mind that big dynamic jumps can damage your joints, so keep it gentle. Repeat this move for 1 minute.

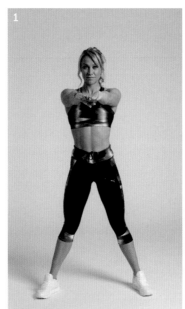

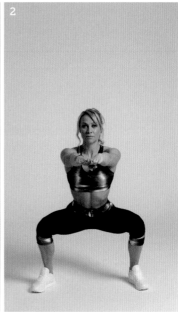

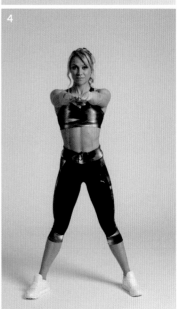

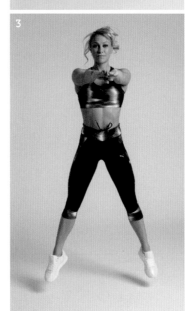

2 SIDE SLIDES x 1 minute

You may need to take your trainers off to do this move or, to save time, find something to stand on that will let your feet slide across the surface, such as a cloth or a cushion. Stand up straight with your feet together and a slight bend in your knees. With your hands clasped together in front of your chest, slide one leg out sideways until it reaches its full extension (within your natural range), while still keeping your foot flat on the ground. Slowly and gently pull your leg back to the centre. Repeat this movement with the opposite leg. Continue alternating your legs for 1 minute.

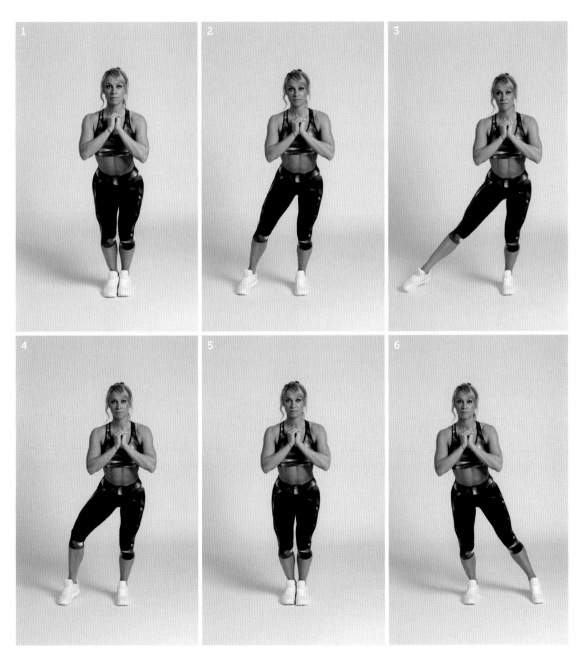

3 LUNGE JUMPS
x 1 minute

Starting in the lunge position with your hands on your hips, jump up quickly and swap leg positions in mid air. Land in the lunge position and then launch straight into the next jump, again switching your feet in mid air. Repeat for the full minute.

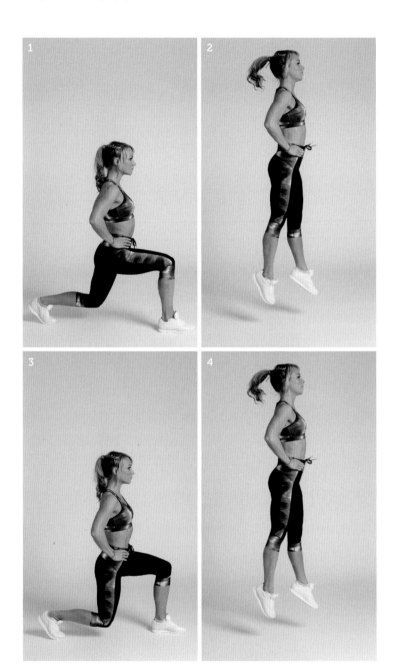

4 HIP THRUSTS x 1 minute

You may need a mat or a soft surface for this exercise. Lie on your back with your feet hip-width apart, knees bent. Slowly and gently thrust your hips up into the air, squeezing your buttocks as you do so. Hold this position for a few seconds before slowly and gently coming back down into your starting position. Repeat this move for the full minute.

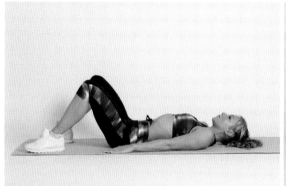 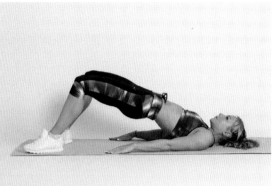

REST x 1 minute

Repeat exercises 1–4 followed by a rest x 6 times
Total: 30 minutes

Cool down
(see pages 43–54)

Monday's Diet:
High Fat, Low Carb

Build your own meals using **only** proteins, fats and non-starchy vegetables – see page 28 for explanation and portion sizes. For recipe ideas on what to have for breakfast, see pages 134–49, choose 2 snacks from the list on page 36 and for recipe ideas on what to have for lunch and dinner, see pages 168–83.

WEEK 1 TUESDAY

WARM UP (see pages 43–54)

EXERCISES 1–4 back to back and then rest for 1 minute
Total: 5 minutes

REPEAT exercises 1–4 followed by a rest x 6 times
Total: 30 minutes

COOL DOWN (see pages 43–54)

1 MOUNTAIN CLIMBERS x 1 minute

Lie on your front, feet hip-width apart, toes facing towards the floor. Place your hands by the sides of your chest, palms facing the floor. Push yourself up by your hands and feet. Bring one knee up to your chest and then back to the starting position. As you do this, switch legs, so you are essentially performing High Knees (see page 108) in a horizontal position. Continue for the full minute.

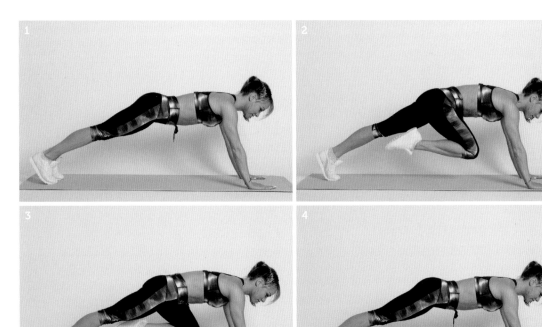

2 V SIT UPS
x 1 minute

You will need a mat or a soft surface for this move. Lie flat on your back, extending your body fully so your arms and legs are outstretched, with only a slight bend in your elbows and knees. Slowly fold your body in on itself, coming up into a V position. Lower your arms until your hands are reaching past your knees. Try to hold this position for a couple of seconds, before slowly and gently returning to your starting position. This movement is quite hard, so you can either get used to it and build up your core strength by speeding it up, or by taking your time. Either way, you eventually want to be able to perform it slowly and fluidly. Repeat this move for 1 minute.

Ab exercises can be very hard for beginners so feel free to make them easier by holding onto something with your hands or feet.

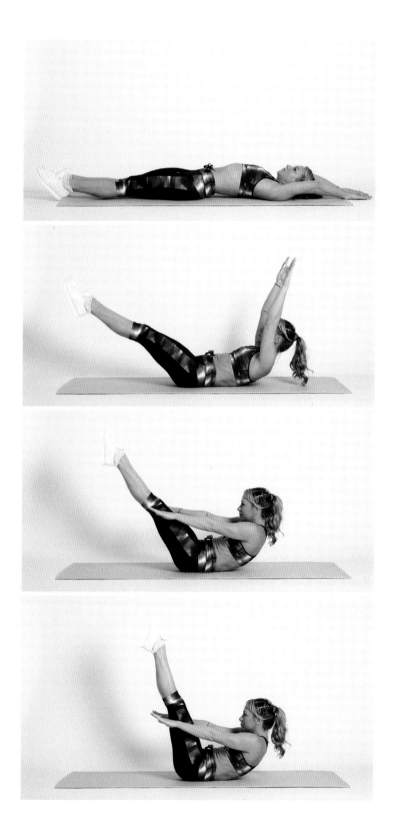

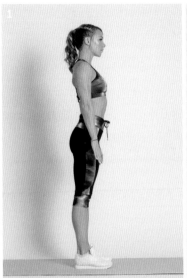

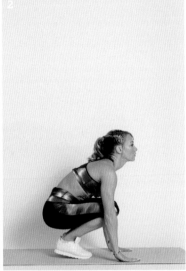

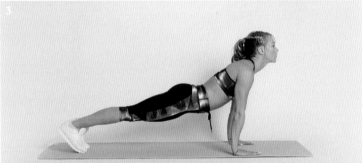

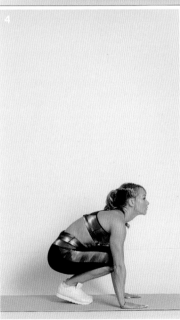

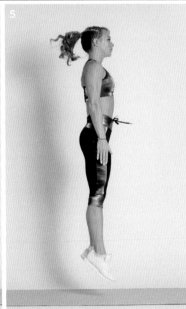

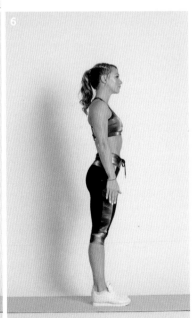

3 BURPEES
x 1 minute

Stand up straight with your feet together and your arms down by your sides. Come down into a crouch (think like a frog) and place your palms flat on the ground in front of you. Put your body weight on your hands and jump your legs backwards, so you are in a hand plank position. Jump your legs back in, knees to your chest, so you return to your crouch position. Explode up into the air in a jump, landing back in your starting position. Repeat this move for the full minute.

4 THE PLANK x 1 minute

You may need a mat or cushion for your elbows during this exercise. Lie on your front with your feet hip-width apart, resting your toes against the top of the mat. Rest on your elbows and keep your forearms flat against the mat. Keep your arms tucked in tight beside you, so your elbows are below your shoulders. Pushing against your toes and forearms, raise your body up into the air, so you form an elevated plank. DO NOT allow your spine to curve, either concavely or convexly. You want a straight back, just like a plank. Try to hold this move for 1 minute. If you are struggling, feel free to transfer your weight from one foot to another, essentially shuffling your feet while holding the plank. Alternatively, come back down on to the mat for a couple of seconds to catch your breath and then return to the plank position to complete the minute.

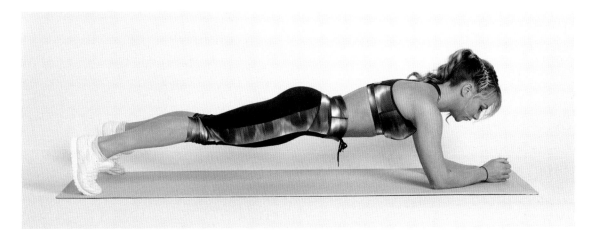

REST x 1 minute

Repeat exercises 1–4 followed by a rest x 6 times Total: 30 minutes

Cool down (see pages 43–54)

Tuesday's Diet:
High Fat, Low Carb

Build your own meals using **only** proteins, fats and non-starchy vegetables – see page 28 for explanation and portion sizes. For recipe ideas on what to have for breakfast, see pages 134–49, choose 2 snacks from the list on page 36 and for recipe ideas on what to have for lunch and dinner, see pages 168–83.

WARM UP
(see pages
43–54)

EXERCISES 1–4
back to back
and then rest
for 1 minute
Total: 5 minutes

REPEAT
exercises 1–4
followed by a rest
x 6 times
Total: 30 minutes

COOL DOWN
(see pages
43–54)

1 MOUNTAIN CLIMBERS x 1 minute

Lie on your front, feet hip-width apart, toes facing towards the floor. Place your hands by the sides of your chest, palms facing the floor. Push yourself up by your hands and feet. Bring one knee up to your chest and then back to the starting position. As you do this, switch legs, so you are essentially performing High Knees (see page 108) in a horizontal position. Continue for the full minute.

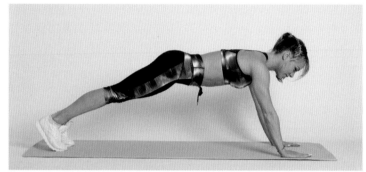

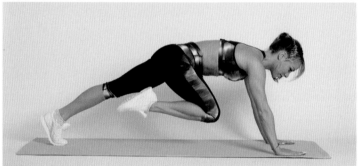

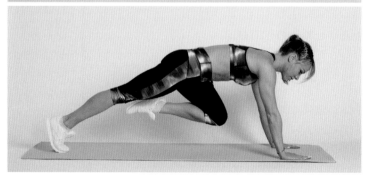

2 TRICEP DIPS
x 1 minute

You will need a chair, a step, a bench, or any slightly raised surface for this movement. Stand facing away from the chair. Place your palms down on the chair and slowly lower your body down by bending at the elbows. Place your legs out in front of you and cross your ankles. Straighten your arms to raise yourself back up into your starting position. Repeat this move for 1 minute. Remember to keep your elbows in tight – they shouldn't be bowing outwards.

Always look at the whole circuit before you begin so you can get everything you need to hand, like a chair for Tricep Dips or a cloth for Side Slides.

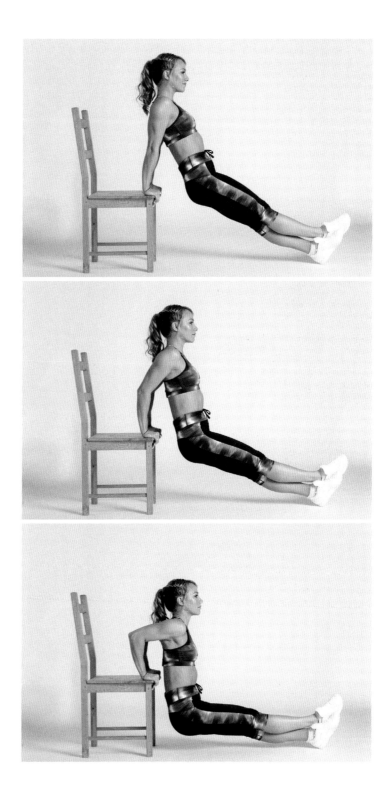

3 WALK OUT PUSH UPS
x 1 minute

Stand up straight with your feet hip-width apart. Allowing your knees to bend slightly, come down and forward out in front of yourself, allowing your hands to touch the floor, palms flat, and place them shoulder-width apart. Crawl outwards until you are fully extended in a horizontal position. Keeping your back straight and bending only at the elbows, perform a push up. Crawl back on yourself until you can stand upright again. Repeat this move for 1 minute.

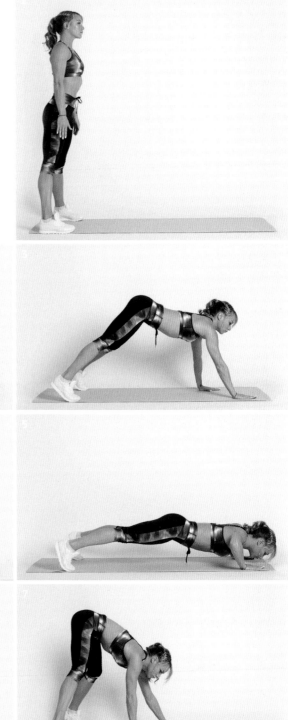

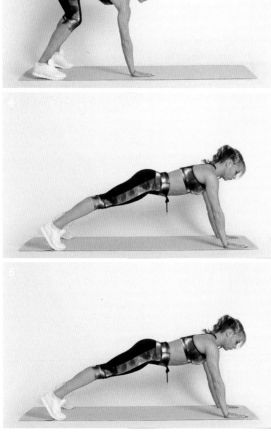

4 ELBOWS TO HAND PLANK x 1 minute

You may need a mat or cushion for your elbows during this exercise. Lie on your front with your feet hip-width apart, resting your toes against the top of the mat. Rest on your elbows and keep your forearms flat against the mat. Keep your arms tucked in tight beside you. Pushing against your toes and forearms, raise your upper body into the air, one arm at a time, to rest on your hands, so you form an elevated plank. DO NOT allow your spine to curve, either concavely or convexly. You need a straight back, just like a plank. Come back down to rest on your forearms and then push back up onto your hands. Repeat this movement for 1 minute.

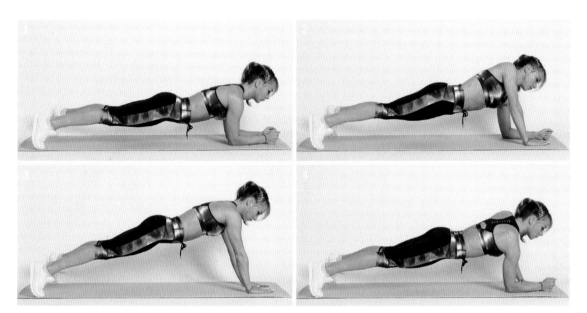

REST x 1 minute

Repeat exercises 1—4 followed by a rest x 6 times Total: 30 minutes

Cool down (see pages 43—54)

Wednesday's Diet:
High Fat, Low Carb

Build your own meals using **only** proteins, fats and non-starchy vegetables – see page 28 for explanation and portion sizes. For recipe ideas on what to have for breakfast, see pages 134–49, choose 2 snacks from the list on page 36 and for recipe ideas on what to have for lunch and dinner, see pages 168–83.

WARM UP (see pages 43–54)

EXERCISES 1–4 back to back and then rest for 1 minute
Total: 5 minutes

REPEAT exercises 1–4 followed by a rest x 6 times
Total: 30 minutes

COOL DOWN (see pages 43–54)

1 STAR JUMPS x 1 minute

Stand up straight with your feet together and your arms down at your sides. Jump your feet outwards (laterally) and, as you do so, bring your arms out and up over your head. Jump back into your starting position and repeat this move for 1 minute. This should be a controlled, fast-paced move.

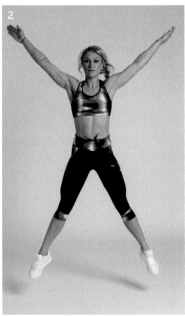

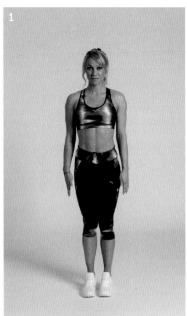

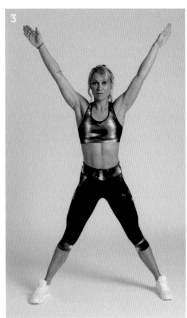

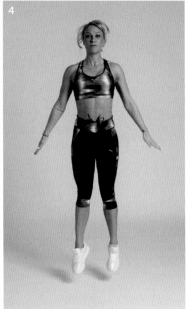

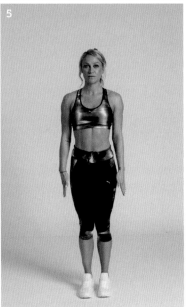

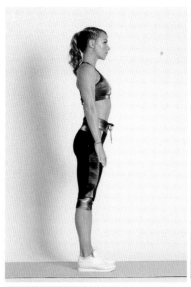

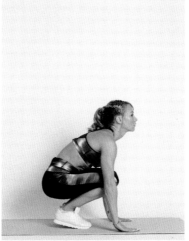

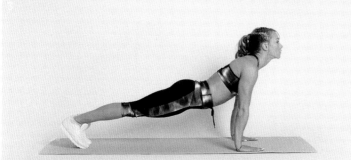

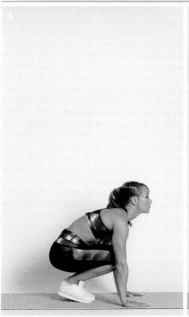

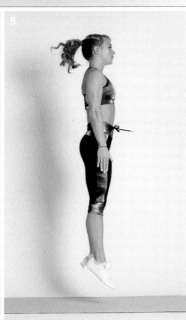

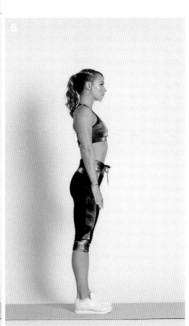

2 BURPEES
x 1 minute

Stand up straight with your feet together and your arms down by your sides. Come down into a crouch (think like a frog) and place your palms flat on the ground in front of you. Put your body weight on your hands and jump your legs backwards, so you are in a hand plank position. Jump your legs back in, knees to your chest, so you return to your crouch position. Explode up into the air in a jump, landing back in your starting position. Repeat this move for the full minute.

3 WALK OUT PUSH UPS
x 1 minute

Stand up straight with your feet hip-width apart. Allowing your knees to bend slightly, come down and forward out in front of yourself, allowing your hands to touch the floor, palms flat, and place them shoulder-width apart. Crawl outwards until you are fully extended in a horizontal position. Keeping your back straight and bending only at the elbows, perform a push up. Crawl back on yourself until you can stand upright again. Repeat this move for 1 minute.

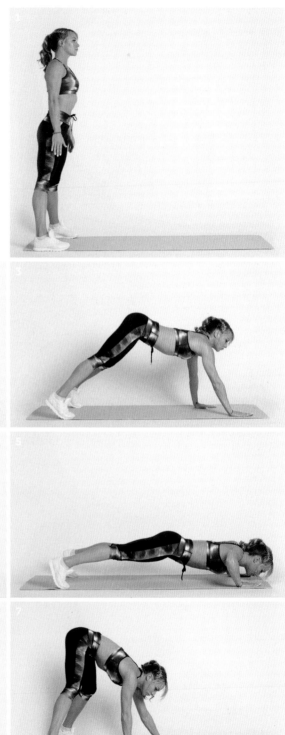

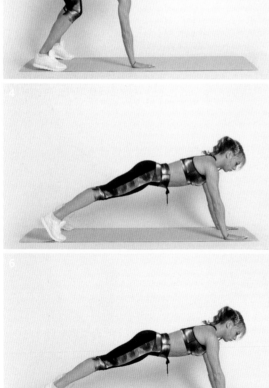

4 MOUNTAIN CLIMBERS
x 1 minute

Lie on your front, feet hip-width apart, toes facing towards the floor. Place your hands by the sides of your chest, palms facing the floor. Push yourself up by your hands and feet. Bring one knee up to your chest and then back to the starting position. As you do this, switch legs, so you are essentially performing High Knees (see page 108) in a horizontal position. Continue for the full minute.

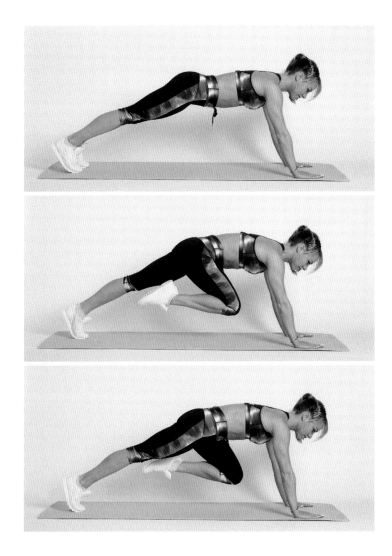

REST x 1 minute

Repeat exercises 1–4 followed by a rest x 6 times
Total: 30 minutes

Cool down
(see pages 43–54)

Thursday's Diet:
High Carb, Low Fat

Build your own meals using **only** proteins, non-starchy vegetables and carbs – see page 28 for explanation and portion sizes. For recipe ideas on what to have for breakfast, see pages 152–64, choose 2 snacks from the list on page 36 and for recipe ideas on what to have for lunch and dinner, see pages 186–99.

WEEK 1 FRIDAY

WARM UP (see pages 43–54)

Perform any circuit of your choice Exercises 1–4 back to back and then rest for 1 minute Total: 5 minutes

REPEAT exercises 1–4 followed by a rest x 6 times Total: 30 minutes

COOL DOWN (see pages 43–54)

Friday's Diet: High Fat, Low Carb

Build your meals using **only** proteins, fats and non-starchy vegetables – see page 28 for explanation and portion sizes. For recipe ideas on what to have for breakfast, see pages 134–49, choose 2 snacks from the list on page 36 and for recipe ideas on what to have for lunch and dinner, see pages 168–83.

WEEK 1 THE WEEKEND

You do not need to train at the weekend. If you feel compelled to, pick a workout of your choice on Saturday – a circuit, a gym class or a leisurely walk – but make sure you have Sunday to rest.

Saturday & Sunday's Diet: High Fat, Low Carb

Build your meals using only proteins, fats and non-starchy vegetables – see page 28 for explanation and portion sizes. For recipe ideas on what to have for breakfast, see pages 134–49, choose 2 snacks from the list on page 36 and for recipe ideas on what to have for lunch and dinner, see pages 168–83.

WEEK
(2)

First and foremost, congratulations
on completing week 1!

HIIT cardio is hard and resistance training is hard, so to
complete 5 very challenging circuits over 5 undoubtedly
gruelling days is something to be proud of. It's not easy,
which is why you've earned some serious respect. Pat
yourself on the back please – you have just won a battle.

Secondly, welcome to week 2...

You'll see that some of the exercises are new and
that I've added another circuit on to each day
(increasing the workout from 30 minutes to 35 minutes,
plus warm up and cool down time).

If you don't want to increase each day's circuit by
5 minutes (perhaps you felt you were at maximum
effort already), you can stick to 5 x 30-minute circuits
and add a 25-minute circuit on day 6 instead
(circuit of your choice). The choice is yours.

Please note: You may struggle to keep going with the
exercise at a dynamic level for the full minute. If this
happens, slow the movement down but don't stop. You
must make sure you complete the entire minute of the
exercise, even if you need to switch to gentle movement.

WARM UP
(see pages
43–54)

EXERCISES 1–4
back to back
and then rest
for 1 minute
Total: 5 minutes

REPEAT
exercises 1–4
followed by a rest
x 7 times
Total: 35 minutes

COOL DOWN
(see pages
43–54)

1 STANDING SQUATS x 1 minute

Stand up straight with your feet hip-width apart. Extend your arms directly out in front of you and place one hand on top of the other – alternatively, place your hands on your hips. Keeping your back straight, lower yourself down into a deep squat by bending your knees. Pushing your weight down against your heels, stand back up straight again. Make sure your knees stay directly above your toes – they shouldn't be collapsing inward. Repeat this move for 1 minute.

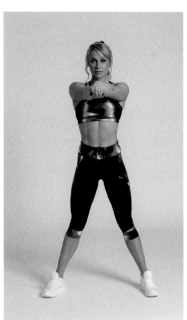
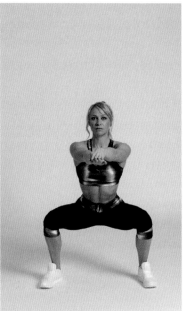
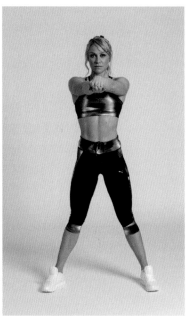

When it comes to squats, form is
very important. Make sure your back stays
straight and your knees stay over your toes.
Engage your core and squat LOW!

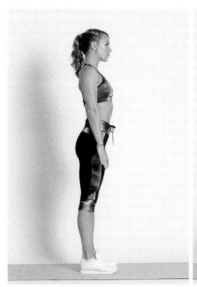

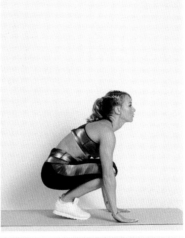

2 BURPEES
x 1 minute

Stand up straight with your feet together and your arms down by your sides. Come down into a crouch (think like a frog) and place your palms flat on the ground in front of you. Put your body weight on your hands and jump your legs backwards, so you are in a hand plank position. Jump your legs back in, knees to your chest, so you return to your crouch position. Explode up into the air in a jump, landing back in your starting position. Repeat this move for the full minute.

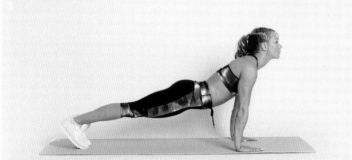

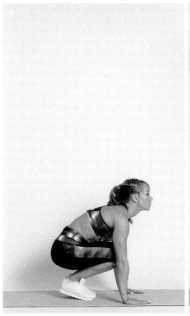

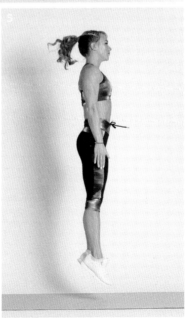

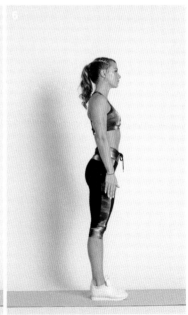

3 DONKEY KICKBACKS x 1 minute

You may need a mat or a soft surface to cushion your knees for this exercise. Get down on your hands and knees so you are on all fours. Make sure to keep your back straight – you don't want to do any damage by arching your spine during this exercise. Keeping the angular bend in your legs at all times, slowly raise one leg up into the air behind you, as far as your natural range will allow, and then 'kick back' further. Hold this position for a second before slowly bringing your leg back down to centre. Repeat the move with the opposite leg and continue to perform alternately for 1 minute.

> You should always engage your glutes and your core. Think about these muscle groups when you perform your exercises.

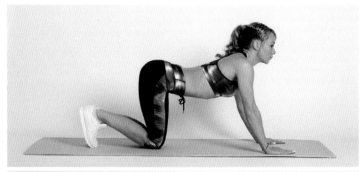

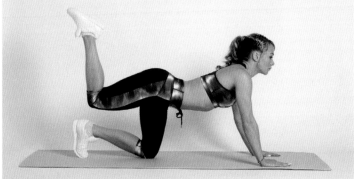

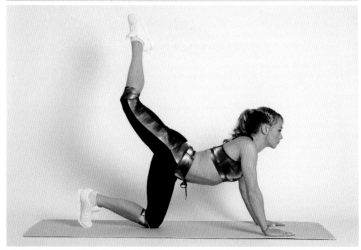

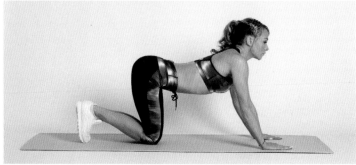

4 INVISIBLE JUMP ROPE x 1 minute

Stand up straight with your feet together, fists out at your sides as if you are about to start skipping. Gently jump up into the air and land softly back down – do this fluidly and rapidly for the full minute.

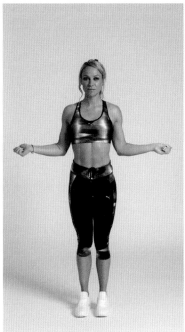
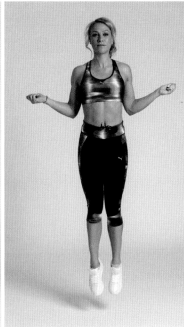
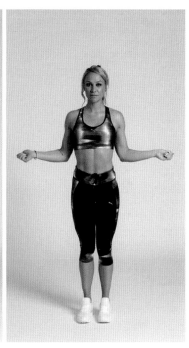

REST x 1 minute

Repeat exercises 1–4 followed by a rest
x 7 times
Total: 35 minutes

Cool down
(see pages 43–54)

Monday's Diet:
High Carb, Low Fat

Build your own meals using **only** proteins, non-starchy vegetables and carbs – see page 28 for explanation and portion sizes. For recipe ideas on what to have for breakfast, see pages 152–64, choose 2 snacks from the list on page 36 and for recipe ideas on what to have for lunch and dinner, see pages 186–99.

WEEK 2 TUESDAY

WARM UP
(see pages
43–54)

EXERCISES 1–4
back to back
and then rest
for 1 minute
Total: 5 minutes

REPEAT
exercises 1–4
followed by a rest
x 7 times
Total: 35 minutes

COOL DOWN
(see pages
43–54)

1 V SIT HOLD
x 1 minute

You will need a mat or a soft surface for this move. Lie flat on your back, extending your body fully so your arms and legs are outstretched, with only a slight bend in your elbows and knees. Slowly fold your body in on itself, coming up into a V position and holding your arms horizontally. Try to maintain this position for 1 minute. If you need to come back down and then repeat the move, you may do so.

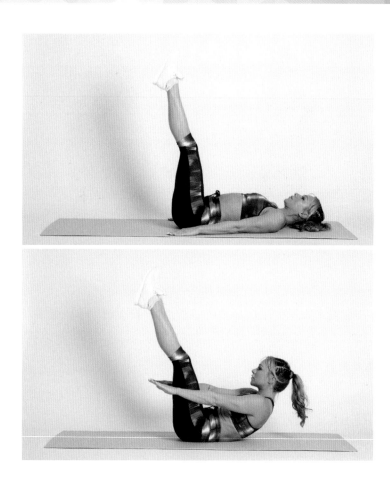

V Sit Holds are hard so if you need
to come back down, do it slowly so your
abs still get a good hit. Take a few breaths
and start again.

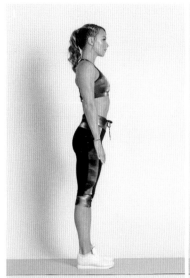
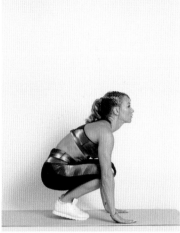

2 BURPEES
x 1 minute

Stand up straight with your feet together and your arms down by your sides. Come down into a crouch (think like a frog) and place your palms flat on the ground in front of you. Put your body weight on your hands and jump your legs backwards, so you are in a hand plank position. Jump your legs back in, knees to your chest, so you return to your crouch position. Explode up into the air in a jump, landing back in your starting position. Repeat this move for the full minute.

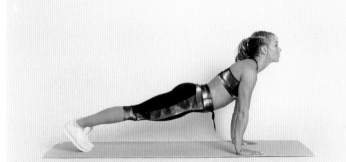

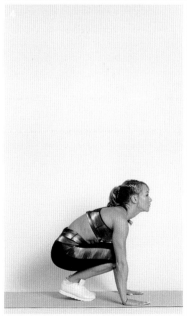
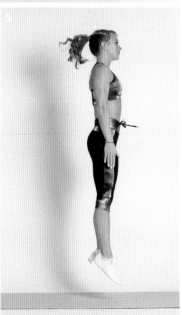
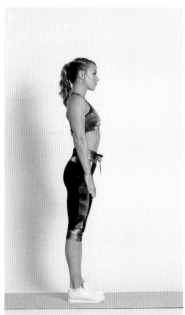

3 SIDE BENDS
x 1 minute

Stand up straight with your feet hip-width apart, your arms flat by your sides, with fingertips pointing down towards the floor. Engaging your core (tensing your mid-section as if you are about to be punched in the stomach), slowly and in a controlled manner, bend to one side as far as your natural range will allow. Still tensing your stomach, use your core to come back up to a straight, standing position (again, slowly and in a controlled manner). Repeat this move on the opposite side. Continue to perform alternately for the full minute.

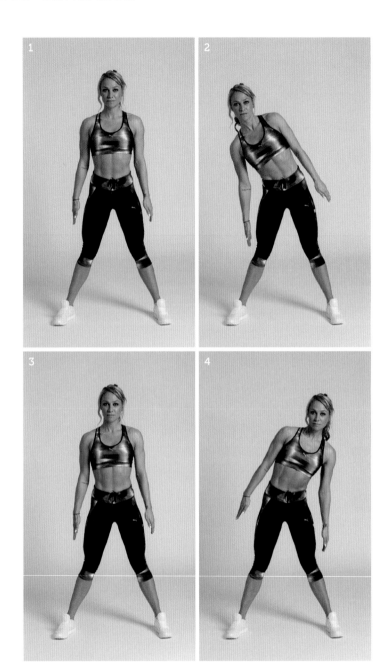

4 WALK OUT PUSH UPS x 1 minute

Stand up straight with your feet hip-width apart. Allowing your knees to bend slightly, come down and forward out in front of yourself, allowing your hands to touch the floor, palms flat, and place them shoulder-width apart. Crawl outwards until you are fully extended in a horizontal position. Keeping your back straight and bending only at the elbows, perform a push up. Crawl back on yourself until you can stand upright again. Repeat this move for 1 minute.

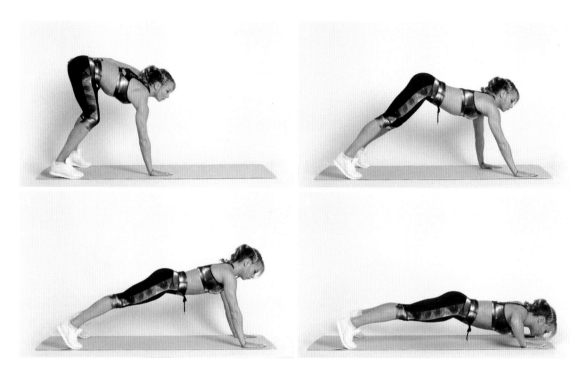

REST x 1 minute

Repeat exercises 1—4 followed by a rest
x 7 times
Total: 35 minutes

Cool down (see pages 43—54)

Tuesday's Diet:
High Fat, Low Carb

Build your own meals using **only** proteins, fats and non-starchy vegetables — see page 28 for explanation and portion sizes. For recipe ideas on what to have for breakfast, see pages 134—49, choose 2 snacks from the list on page 36 and for recipe ideas on what to have for lunch and dinner, see pages 168—83.

WARM UP
(see pages
43–54)

EXERCISES 1–4
back to back
and then rest
for 1 minute
Total: 5 minutes

REPEAT
exercises 1–4
followed by a rest
x 7 times
Total: 35 minutes

COOL DOWN
(see pages
43–54)

1 WALL PUSHES x 1 minute

Find a bare wall and stand in front of it, feet hip-width apart. Place your palms flat against the wall, shoulder-width apart. Keeping your back straight and bending only at the elbows, perform a vertical push up against the wall. As you push back, give a very gentle push, and allow yourself to fall back on to the wall into your starting position. Repeat this move for 1 minute.

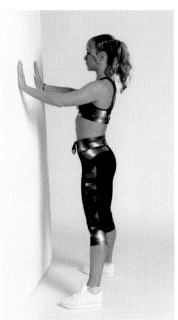
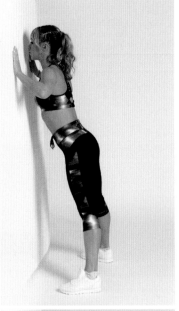
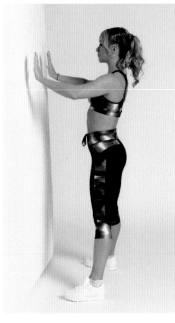
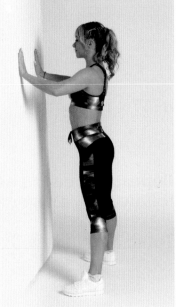

2 STAR JUMPS
x 1 minute

Stand up straight with your feet together and your arms down at your sides. Jump your feet outwards (laterally) and, as you do so, bring your arms out and up over your head. Jump back into your starting position and repeat this move for 1 minute. This should be a controlled, fast-pace move.

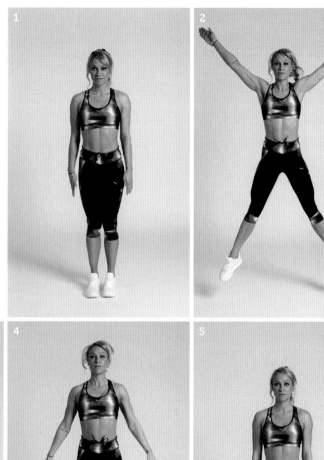

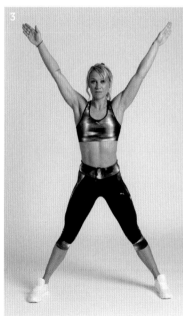

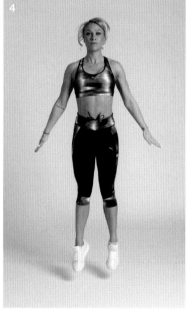

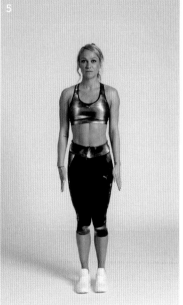

Really concentrate on using your upper body strength in the Wall Pushes to lower yourself against, and slowly push yourself back from, the wall.

3 PUSH UPS x 1 minute

Stand up straight with your feet hip-width apart. Allowing your knees to bend slightly, come down and forward out in front of yourself, allowing your hands to touch the floor, palms flat, placed shoulder-width apart. Crawl outwards until you are fully extended in a horizontal position. Keeping your back straight, bending only at the elbows, perform a push up. Repeat this move for 1 minute. If you need to come on to your knees to complete the full minute, you may do so.

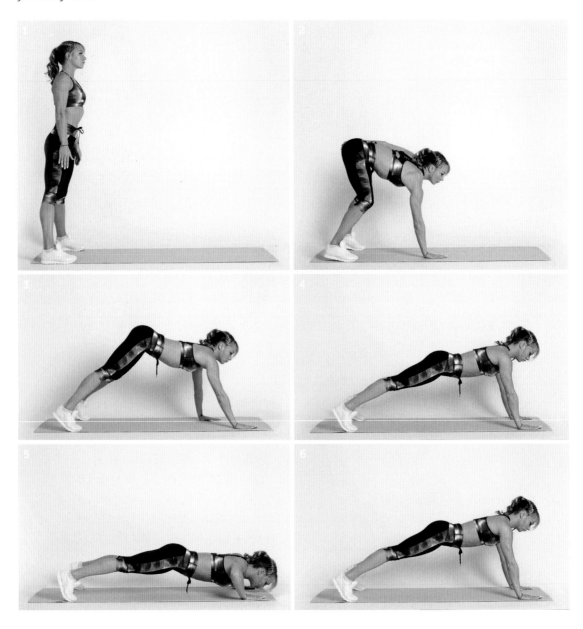

4 INVISIBLE JUMP ROPE x 1 minute

Stand up straight with your feet together, fists out at your sides as if you are about to start skipping. Gently jump up into the air and land softly back down – do this fluidly and rapidly for the full minute.

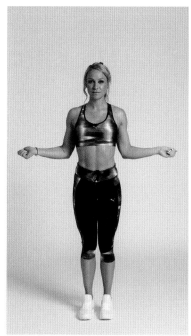
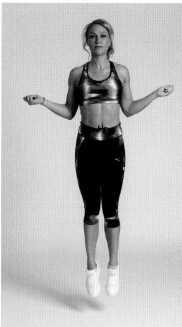
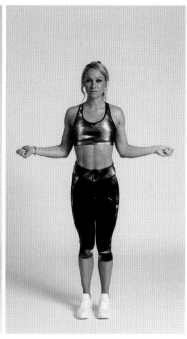

REST x 1 minute

Repeat exercises 1–4 followed by a rest
x 7 times
Total: 35 minutes

Cool down (see pages 43–54)

Wednesday's Diet:
High Fat, Low Carb

Build your own meals using **only** proteins, fats and non-starchy vegetables – see page 28 for explanation and portion sizes. For recipe ideas on what to have for breakfast, see pages 134–49, choose 2 snacks from the list on page 36 and for recipe ideas on what to have for lunch and dinner, see pages 168–83.

WEEK 2 THURSDAY

WARM UP (see pages 43–54)

EXERCISES 1–4 back to back and then rest for 1 minute
Total: 5 minutes

REPEAT exercises 1–4 followed by a rest x 7 times
Total: 35 minutes

COOL DOWN (see pages 43–54)

1 SQUAT JUMPS x 1 minute

Stand up straight with your feet hip-width apart. Extend your arms directly out in front of you and place one hand on top of the other – alternatively, place your hands on your hips. Keeping your back straight, lower yourself down into a deep squat by bending your knees. Instead of standing back up again from the squat, gently jump back into a standing position. The jump should be so gentle that you can maintain your form from the very start of the exercise to the next repetition. It should also be so gentle that you only come off the floor a little. Bear in mind that big dynamic jumps can damage your joints, so keep it gentle. Repeat this move for 1 minute.

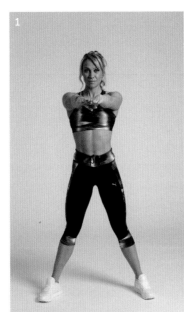
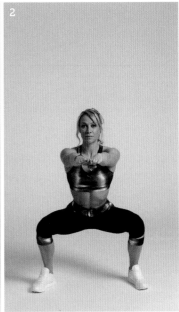
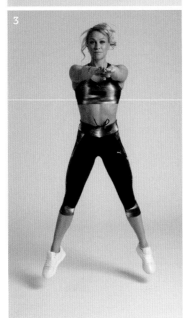
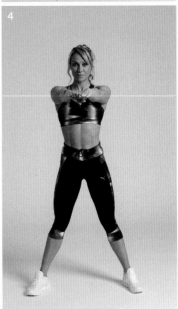

2 INVISIBLE JUMP ROPE x 1 minute

Stand up straight with your feet together, fists out at your sides as if you are about to start skipping. Gently jump up into the air and land softly back down – do this fluidly and rapidly for the full minute.

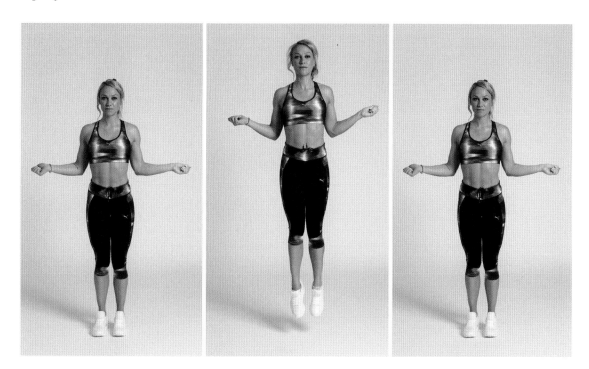

Even though the rope is invisible, you still need to jump as if it's there. Don't give yourself an easy ride – push yourself!

3 LUNGE JUMPS
x 1 minute

Starting in the lunge position with your hands on your hips, jump up quickly and swap leg positions in mid air. Land in the lunge position and then launch straight into the next jump, again switching your feet in mid air. Repeat for the full minute.

I don't want you jumping like a crazed kangaroo – it's not good for your tendons or your joints! Jump enough to do the exercise but do so in a contolled and gentle manner.

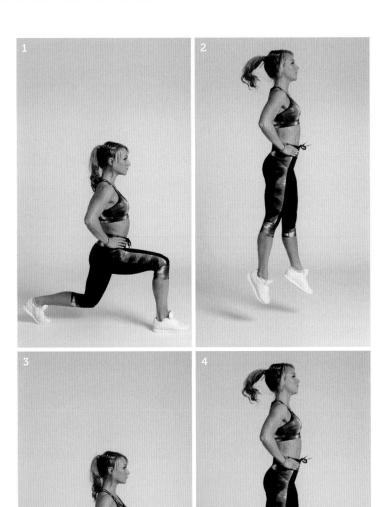

4 ELBOWS TO HAND PLANK x 1 minute

You may need a mat or cushion for your elbows during this exercise. Lie on your front with your feet hip-width apart, resting your toes against the top of the mat. Rest on your elbows and keep your forearms flat against the mat. Keep your arms tucked in tight beside you. Pushing against your toes and forearms, raise your upper body into the air, one arm at a time, to rest on your hands, so you form an elevated plank. DO NOT allow your spine to curve, either concavely or convexly. You need a straight back, just like a plank. Come back down to rest on your forearms and then push back up onto your hands. Repeat this movement for 1 minute.

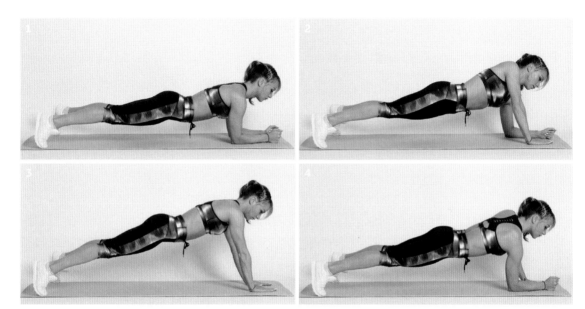

REST x 1 minute

Repeat exercises 1–4 followed by a rest
x 7 times
Total: 35 minutes

Cool down (see pages 43–54)

Thursday's Diet:
High Fat, Low Carb

Build your own meals using **only** proteins, fats and non-starchy vegetables – see page 28 for explanation and portion sizes. For recipe ideas on what to have for breakfast, see pages 134–49, choose 2 snacks from the list on page 36 and for recipe ideas on what to have for lunch and dinner, see pages 168–83.

WEEK 2 FRIDAY

WARM UP
(see pages 43–54)

Perform any circuit of your choice
Exercises 1–4 back to back and then rest for 1 minute
Total: 5 minutes

REPEAT
exercises 1–4 followed by a rest x 7 times
Total: 35 minutes

COOL DOWN
(see pages 43–54)

Friday's Diet: High Carb, Low Fat

Build your meals using **only** proteins, non-starchy vegetables and carbs – see page 28 for explanation and portion sizes. For recipe ideas on what to have for breakfast, see pages 152–64, choose 2 snacks from the list on page 36 and for recipe ideas on what to have for lunch and dinner, see pages 186–99.

WEEK 2 THE WEEKEND

If you managed to do the 35-minute circuits, then you don't need to train at the weekend, unless you feel compelled to. If you do, pick any of the week's workouts for Saturday but make sure you have Sunday to rest.

If you decided to keep to 30-minute circuits on Monday–Friday, don't forget to do a 25-minute circuit on Saturday.

Saturday & Sunday's Diet: High Fat, Low Carb

Build your meals using only proteins, fats and non-starchy vegetables – see page 28 for explanation and portion sizes. For recipe ideas on what to have for breakfast, see pages 134–49, choose 2 snacks from the list on page 36 and for recipe ideas on what to have for lunch and dinner, see pages 168–83.

WEEK

Congratulations, you're now
officially at the half-way point!

**Now is the time to PUSH in order to get
the best results possible.**

**You'll see that some of the exercises are new and
that I've added another circuit on to each day
(increasing the workout from 35 minutes to 40 minutes,
plus warm up and cool down time).**

**If you don't want to increase each day's circuit by
5 minutes (perhaps you stuck with the 30-minute
circuits in week 2 and want to try 35 minutes this week,
rather than jumping to 40 minutes), you can stick
to 35-minute circuits and add a 25-minute circuit
on to day 6 instead (circuit of your choice).
It's entirely up to you.**

Please note: You may struggle to keep going with
the exercise at a dynamic level for the full minute.
If this happens, slow the movement down but don't stop.
You must make sure you complete the entire minute of the
exercise, even if you need to switch to gentle movement.

WARM UP
(see pages
43–54)

EXERCISES 1–4
back to back
and then rest
for 1 minute
Total: 5 minutes

REPEAT
exercises 1–4
followed by a rest
x 8 times
Total: 40 minutes

COOL DOWN
(see pages
43–54)

1 DONKEY SIDE KICKS x 1 minute

You may need a mat or a soft surface to cushion your knees for this exercise. Get down on your hands and knees so you are on all fours. Make sure you keep your back straight – you don't want to do any damage by arching your spine during this exercise. Keeping the angular bend in your legs at all times, slowly raise one leg up and out to the side, until you feel the tension in your buttocks. Hold this position for 1 second before slowly bringing your leg back down to the centre. Repeat with the opposite leg and continue to perform the move alternately for 1 minute.

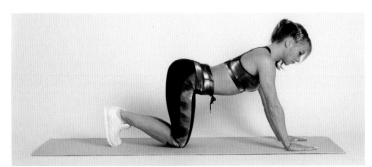

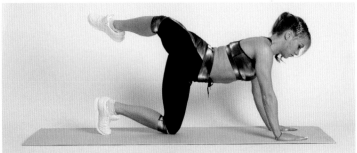

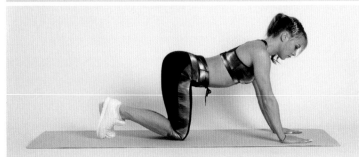

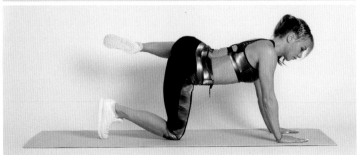

2 STAR JUMPS
x 1 minute

Stand up straight with your feet together and your arms down at your sides. Jump your feet outwards (laterally) and, as you do so, bring your arms out and up over your head. Jump back into your starting position and repeat this move for 1 minute. This should be a controlled, fast-pace move.

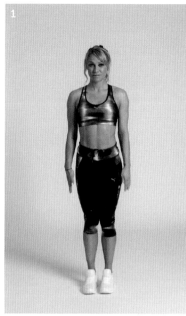
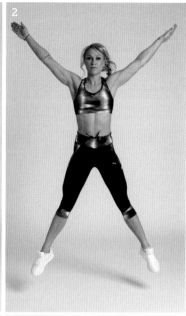
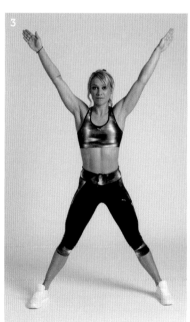
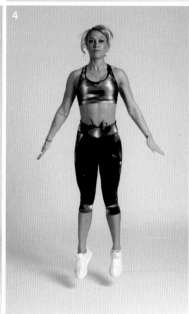
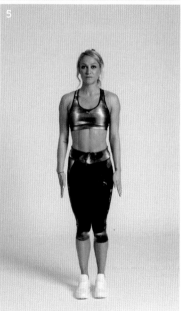

3 ALTERNATE LUNGES
x 1 minute

Stand up straight with your feet together and your hands on your hips. Lunge forward with one leg, as far as your natural range will allow. Bending your knees, come down into the lunge, allowing your back knee to hover just above floor level and keeping your front knee directly above your toes. Push back up into your starting position and repeat with the opposite leg. Perform alternately for 1 minute.

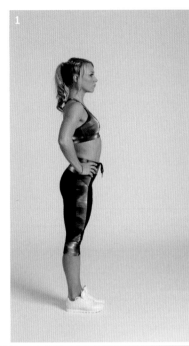

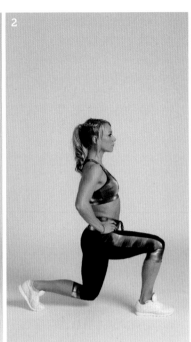

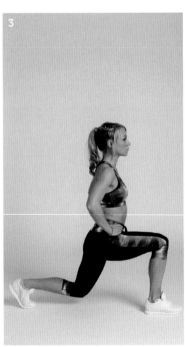

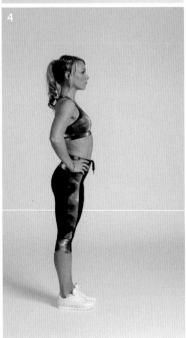

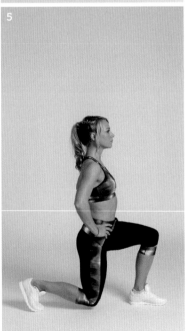

4 MOUNTAIN CLIMBERS
x 1 minute

Lie on your front, feet hip-width apart, toes facing towards the floor. Place your hands by the sides of your chest, palms facing the floor. Push yourself up by your hands and feet. Bring one knee up to your chest and then back to the starting position. As you do this, switch legs, so you are essentially performing High Knees (see page 108) in a horizontal position. Continue for the full minute.

REST x 1 minute

Repeat exercises 1–4 followed by a rest
x 8 times
Total: 40 minutes

Cool down
(see pages 43–54)

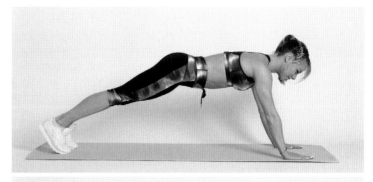

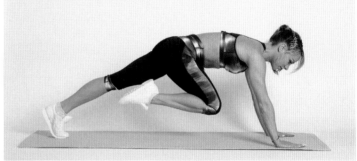

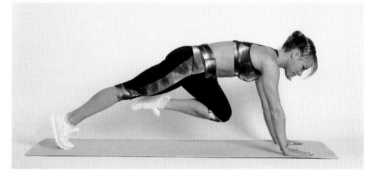

Monday's Diet:
High Fat, Low Carb

Build your own meals using **only** proteins, fats and non-starchy vegetables – see page 28 for explanation and portion sizes. For recipe ideas on what to have for breakfast, see pages 134–49, choose 2 snacks from the list on page 36 and for recipe ideas on what to have for lunch and dinner, see pages 168–83.

WEEK 3 TUESDAY

WARM UP (see pages 43–54)

EXERCISES 1–4 back to back and then rest for 1 minute
Total: 5 minutes

REPEAT exercises 1–4 followed by a rest x 8 times
Total: 40 minutes

COOL DOWN (see pages 43–54)

1 RUSSIAN TWISTS x 1 minute

You will need a mat or a soft surface for this move. Sit down on the mat and place your legs out in front of you with a slight bend in your knees. Cross your ankles and slowly raise your heels a little off the ground. You want to keep your lower body in this exact position throughout the exercise – the only thing that should be moving is a slight twist in your core, followed through with your upper body. Place your hands out in front of you and clasp them together. Twist your core to one side, moving your hands along with it. When the twist is complete, immediately continue the move to the opposite side. This should be a fluid movement, twisting from one side to the other, repeated for the full minute. If you find this movement too trying at first, build up your core strength initially by keeping your heels on the floor and performing the twist in your core and upper body alone. However, you must aim to achieve the twist with your feet raised off the ground.

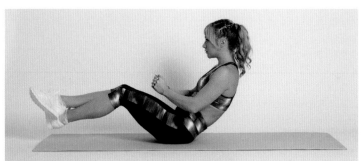
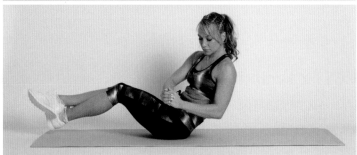
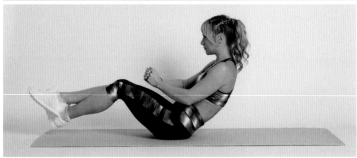
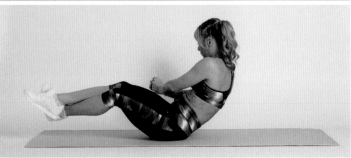

2 INVISIBLE JUMP ROPE x 1 minute

Stand up straight with your feet together, fists out at your sides as if you are about to start skipping. Gently jump up into the air and land softly back down – do this fluidly and rapidly for the full minute.

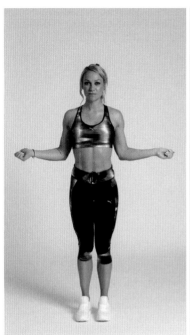 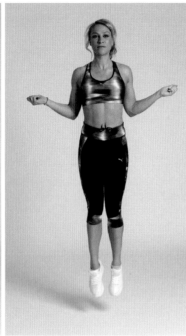 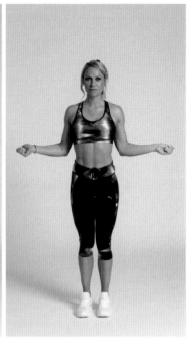

Core exercises, like Russian Twists, can be hard for beginners. If you need to alter the movement slightly, you may do so.

3 LEG RAISES
x 1 minute

You will need a mat or a soft surface for this move. Lie flat on your back, extending your legs out fully and crossing your ankles. Keep your arms flat by your sides – feel free to hold onto the sides of the mat or onto a solid object (like a sofa or a table) behind your head to make this move easier. Slowly raise your legs up into the air so they are vertical above your body, give a little upward thrust with your hips, raising your bottom off the floor, and then slowly bring your legs back down to just above ground level. Repeat this movement for the full minute.

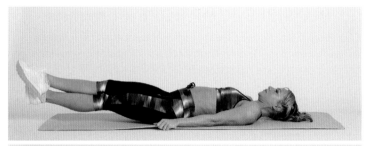

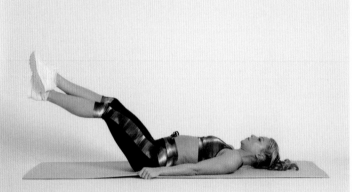

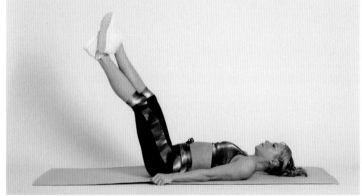

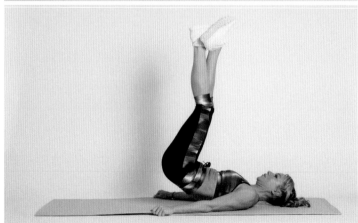

4 LUNGE JUMPS x 1 minute

Starting in the lunge position with your hands on your hips, jump up quickly and swap leg positions in mid air. Land in the lunge position and then launch straight into the next jump, again switching your feet in mid air. Repeat for the full minute.

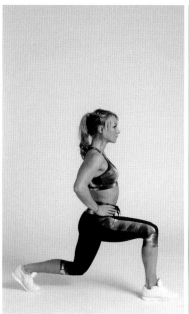
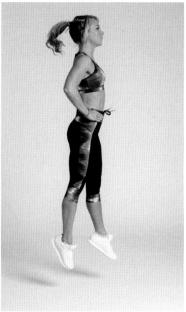
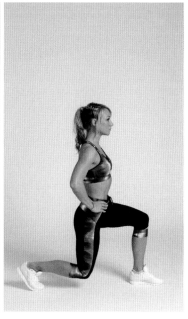

REST x 1 minute

Repeat exercises 1–4 followed by a rest
x 8 times
Total: 40 minutes

Cool down
(see pages 43–54)

Tuesday's Diet:
High Fat, Low Carb

Build your own meals using **only** proteins, fats and non-starchy vegetables – see page 28 for explanation and portion sizes. For recipe ideas on what to have for breakfast, see pages 134–49, choose 2 snacks from the list on page 36 and for recipe ideas on what to have for lunch and dinner, see pages 168–83.

WARM UP
(see pages 43–54)

EXERCISES 1–4
back to back
and then rest
for 1 minute
Total: 5 minutes

REPEAT
exercises 1–4
followed by a rest
x 8 times
Total: 40 minutes

COOL DOWN
(see pages 43–54)

1 THE PLANK x 1 minute

You may need a mat or cushion for your elbows during this exercise. Lie on your front with your feet hip-width apart, resting your toes against the top of the mat. Rest on your elbows and keep your forearms flat against the mat. Keep your arms tucked in tight beside you, so your elbows are below your shoulders. Pushing against your toes and forearms, raise your body up into the air, so you form an elevated plank. DO NOT allow your spine to curve, either concavely or convexly. You want a straight back, just like a plank. Try to hold this move for 1 minute. If you are struggling, feel free to transfer your weight from one foot to another, essentially shuffling your feet while holding the plank. Alternatively, come back down on to the mat for a couple of seconds to catch your breath and then return to the plank position to complete the minute.

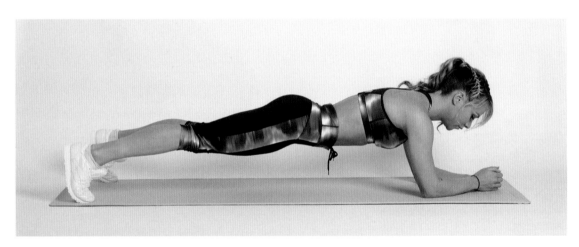

You will find you get better at
The Plank as your core strength increases.
Always aim to improve every week.

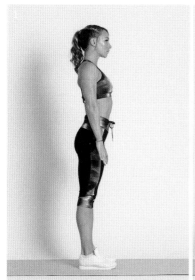
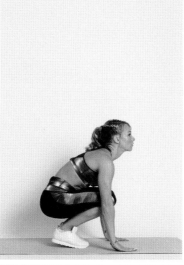
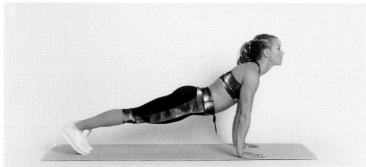

2 BURPEES
x 1 minute

Stand up straight with your feet together and your arms down by your sides. Come down into a crouch (think like a frog) and place your palms flat on the ground in front of you. Put your body weight on your hands and jump your legs backwards, so you are in a hand plank position. Jump your legs back in, knees to your chest, so you return to your crouch position. Explode up into the air in a jump, landing back in your starting position. Repeat this move for the full minute.

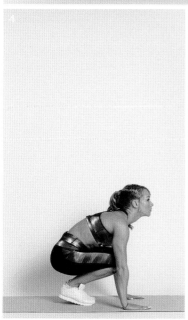
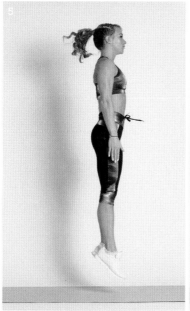
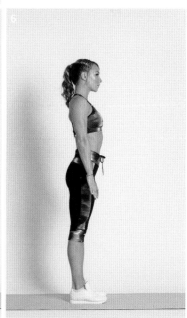

3 DIAMOND PUSH UPS x 1 minute

Stand up straight with your feet hip-width apart. Allowing your knees to bend slightly, come down and forward in front of yourself, allowing your hands to touch the floor, palms flat, thumbs and forefingers touching to form a diamond shape. Keeping your back straight and bending only at the elbows, perform a push up. Repeat this move for 1 minute. If you need to come onto your knees to complete the full minute, you may do so.

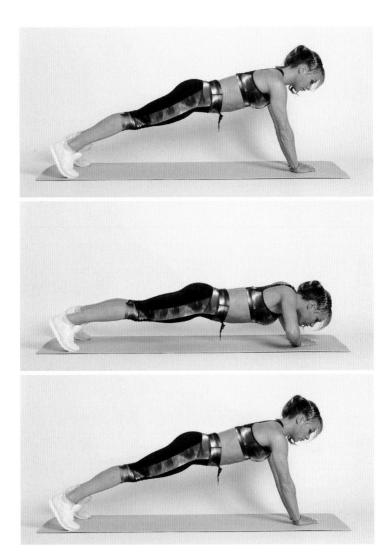

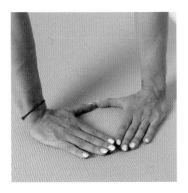

Regular Push Ups will hit your chest but Diamond Push Ups target your triceps, aka your 'bingo wings'!

4 WALK OUT PUSH UPS x 1 minute

Stand up straight with your feet hip-width apart. Allowing your knees to bend slightly, come down and forward out in front of yourself, allowing your hands to touch the floor, palms flat, and place them shoulder-width apart. Crawl outwards until you are fully extended in a horizontal position. Keeping your back straight and bending only at the elbows, perform a push up. Crawl back on yourself until you can stand upright again. Repeat this move for 1 minute.

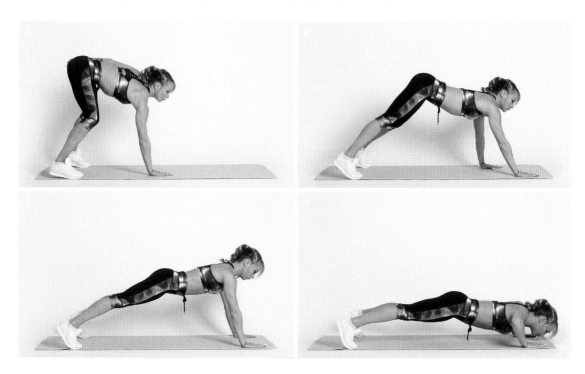

REST x 1 minute

Repeat exercises 1–4 followed by a rest
x 8 times
Total: 40 minutes

Cool down (see pages 43–54)

Wednesday's Diet:
High Carb, Low Fat

Build your own meals using **only** proteins, non-starchy vegetables and carbs – see page 28 for explanation and portion sizes. For recipe ideas on what to have for breakfast, see pages 152–64, choose 2 snacks from the list on page 36 and for recipe ideas on what to have for lunch and dinner, see pages 186–99.

| WARM UP (see pages 43–54) | EXERCISES 1–4 back to back and then rest for 1 minute Total: 5 minutes | REPEAT exercises 1–4 followed by a rest x 8 times Total: 40 minutes | COOL DOWN (see pages 43–54) |

1 INVISIBLE JUMP ROPE x 1 minute

Stand up straight with your feet together, fists out at your sides as if you are about to start skipping. Gently jump up into the air and land softly back down – do this fluidly and rapidly for the full minute.

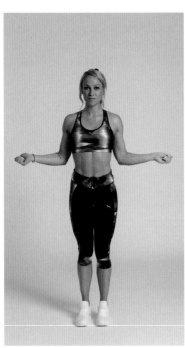
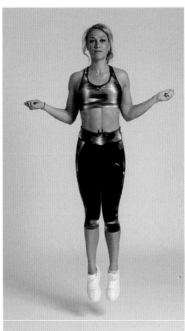
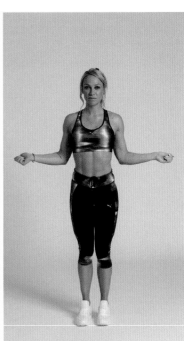

This is a very cardiovascular circuit so really give it 100% and BURN THAT FAT!

2 ON THE SPOTS
x 1 minute

Stand up straight with
your feet together. Run
on the spot as fast as you
can, punching the air with
your hands. Continue this
move for 1 minute.

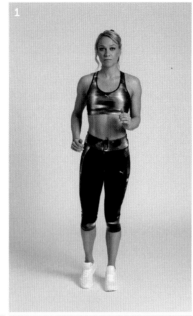

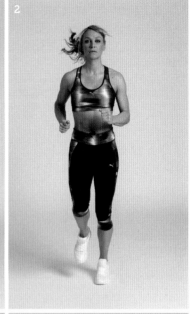

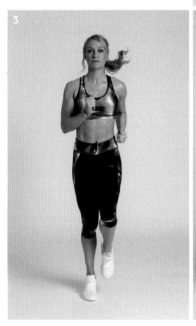

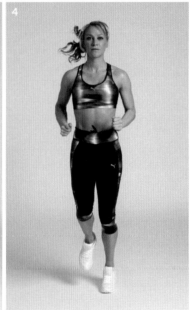

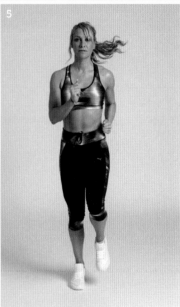

3 HIGH KNEES x 1 minute

Stand up straight with your feet together. Break into an on-the-spot sprint, raising your knees as high as you can and punching the air with your fists. Perform this move intensely for the full minute.

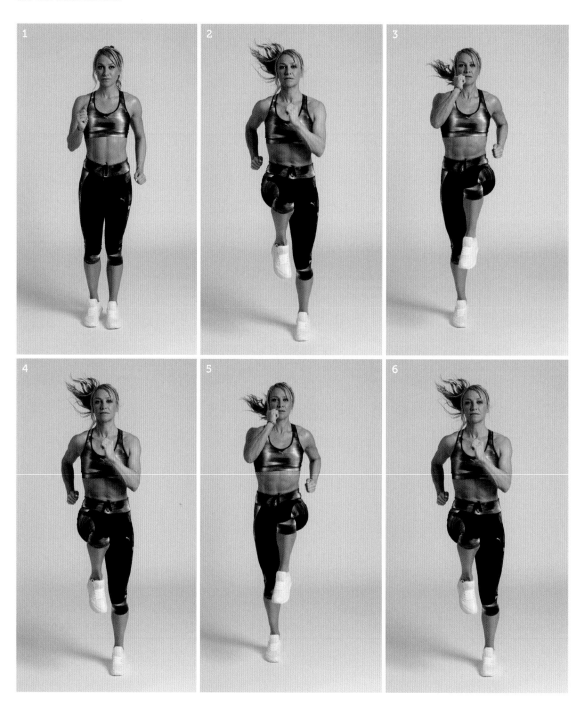

4 INVISIBLE SIDE SKIPS x 1 minute

Stand up straight with your feet together, fists out at your sides as if you are about to start skipping. Gently jump up and to one side and then land softly back down, before immediately jumping to the opposite side. Switch from side to side like this fluidly and rapidly for the full minute.

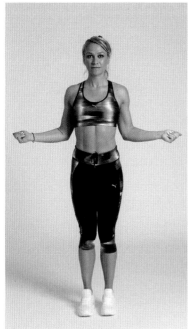
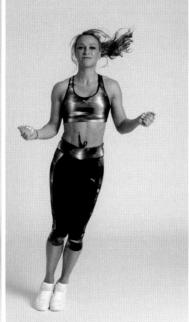
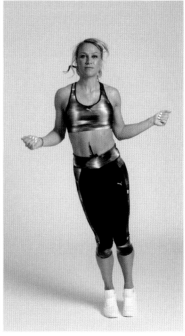

REST x 1 minute

Repeat exercises 1—4 followed by a rest
x 8 times
Total: 40 minutes

Cool down
(see pages 43—54)

Thursday's Diet:
High Fat, Low Carb

Build your own meals using **only** proteins, fats and non-starchy vegetables — see page 28 for explanation and portion sizes. For recipe ideas on what to have for breakfast, see pages 134—49, choose 2 snacks from the list on page 36 and for recipe ideas on what to have for lunch and dinner, see pages 168—83.

WEEK 3 FRIDAY

WARM UP (see pages 43–54)

Perform any circuit of your choice **Exercises 1–4 back to back and then rest for 1 minute** Total: 5 minutes

REPEAT exercises 1–4 followed by a rest x 8 times Total: 40 minutes

COOL DOWN (see pages 43–54)

Friday's Diet: High Fat, Low Carb

Build your meals using **only** proteins, fats and non-starchy vegetables – see page 28 for explanation and portion sizes. For recipe ideas on what to have for breakfast, see pages 134–49, choose 2 snacks from the list on page 36 and for recipe ideas on what to have for lunch and dinner, see pages 168–83.

WEEK 3 THE WEEKEND

If you managed to do the 40-minute circuits, then you don't need to train at the weekend, unless you feel compelled to. If you do, pick any of the week's workouts for Saturday but make sure you have Sunday to rest.

If you decided to keep to 35-minute circuits on Monday–Friday, don't forget to do a 25-minute circuit on Saturday.

Saturday and Sunday's Diet: High Fat, Low Carb

Build your meals using **only** proteins, fats and non-starchy vegetables – see page 28 for explanation and portion sizes. For recipe ideas on what to have for breakfast, see pages 134–49, choose 2 snacks from the list on page 36 and for recipe ideas on what to have for lunch and dinner, see pages 168–83.

WEEK

(4)

Congratulations on making it to the final week!

By week 4 your body is probably a bit tired and your brain is probably a bit fed up.

But now is NOT the time to quit!

Now is the time to PUSH!

You have 1 week left to get THE BEST RESULTS POSSIBLE!

You'll see that some of the exercises are new and I've added another day of training on Saturday, so you'll now be doing 6 x 40-minute circuits.

Please note: You may struggle to keep going with the exercise at a dynamic level for the full minute. If this happens, slow the movement down but don't stop. You must make sure you complete the entire minute of the exercise, even if you need to switch to gentle movement.

WARM UP
(see pages 43–54)

EXERCISES 1–4
back to back and then rest for 1 minute
Total: 5 minutes

REPEAT
exercises 1–4 followed by a rest x 8 times
Total: 40 minutes

COOL DOWN
(see pages 43–54)

1 SIDE LUNGES x 1 minute

Stand up straight with your feet together. With your hands clasped together in front of your chest, take a big step out to one side with your right leg. Once you have planted your right foot on the floor, bend your left knee and come down into a side lunge. This will stretch out your right leg. Once you have come down as far as you can (within your natural range), push yourself back into your initial standing position. Repeat this movement with the opposite leg. Continue to perform alternately for the full minute.

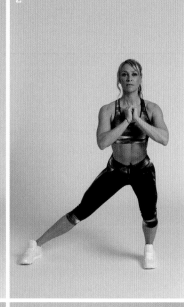

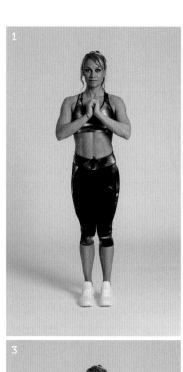

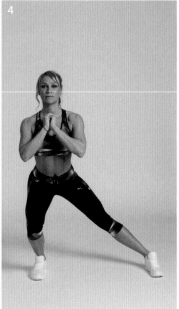

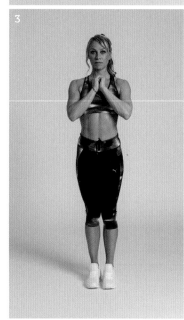

2 SQUAT JUMPS x 1 minute

Stand up straight with your feet hip-width apart. Extend your arms directly out in front of you and place one hand on top of the other – alternatively, place your hands on your hips. Keeping your back straight, lower yourself down into a deep squat by bending your knees. Instead of standing back up again from the squat, gently jump back into a standing position. The jump should be so gentle that you can maintain your form from the very start of the exercise to the next repetition. It should also be so gentle that you only come off the floor a little. Bear in mind that big dynamic jumps can damage your joints, so keep it gentle. Repeat this move for 1 minute.

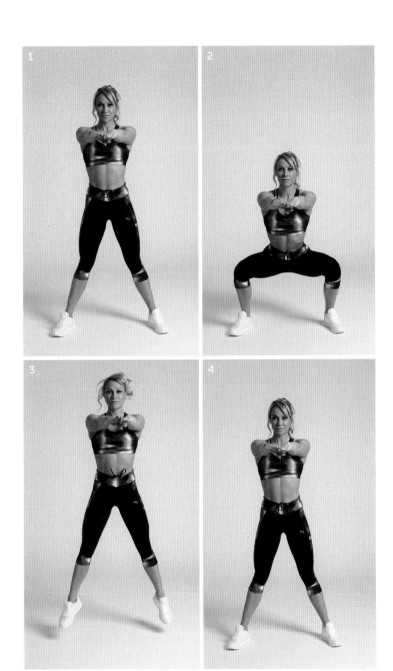

3 KNEE OUTS
x 1 minute

Stand up straight with your feet hip-width apart and your hands clasped together in front of you. Come down into a low squat – as low as your natural range will allow. Extend your knees out to the sides and then bring them back to the centre again. Squeeze your buttocks as you do this. Repeat for the full minute.

There are different ways of doing this exercise – however you feel comfortable while also hitting your glutes is fine.

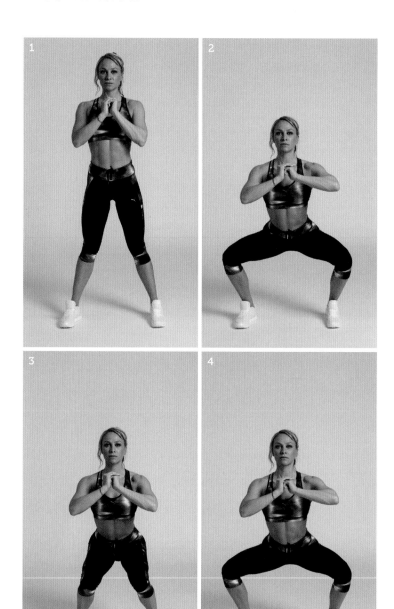

4 LUNGE JUMPS x 1 minute

Starting in the lunge position with your hands on your hips, jump up quickly and swap leg positions in mid air. Land in the lunge position and then launch straight into the next jump, again switching your feet in mid air. Repeat for the full minute.

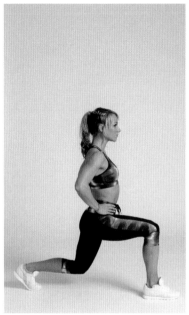
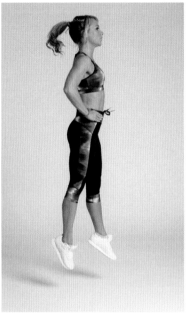
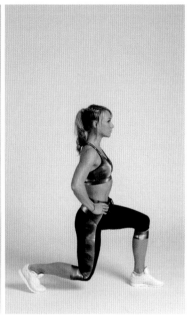

REST x 1 minute

Repeat exercises 1–4 followed by a rest
x 8 times
Total: 40 minutes

Cool down
(see pages 43–54)

Monday's Diet:
High Carb, Low Fat

Build your own meals using **only** proteins, non-starchy vegetables and carbs – see page 28 for explanation and portion sizes. For recipe ideas on what to have for breakfast, see pages 152–64, choose 2 snacks from the list on page 36 and for recipe ideas on what to have for lunch and dinner, see pages 186–99.

WEEK 4 TUESDAY

WARM UP (see pages 43–54)

EXERCISES 1–4 back to back and then rest for 1 minute
Total: 5 minutes

REPEAT exercises 1–4 followed by a rest x 8 times
Total: 40 minutes

COOL DOWN (see pages 43–54)

1 SIDE PLANK x 1 minute

You may need a mat or cushion for this exercise. Lie down on your side and prop your upper body up on your forearm (with a cushion underneath, if desired). Raise your outside hip up into the air and simultaneously push against your forearm and feet. Once one side of your body is raised into the air in a rigid, straight line, engage your core and hold this position for half a minute. Change sides and hold for the remainder of the minute.

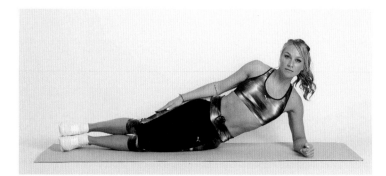

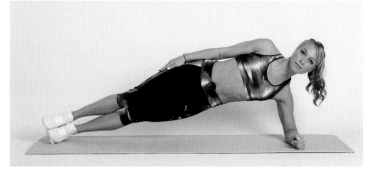

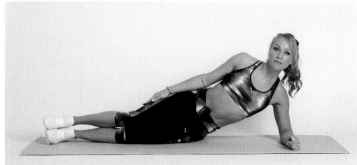

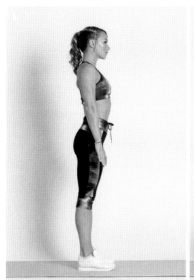

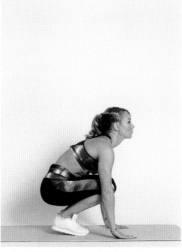

2 BURPEES x 1 minute

Stand up straight with your feet together and your arms down by your sides. Come down into a crouch (think like a frog) and place your palms flat on the ground in front of you. Put your body weight on your hands and jump your legs backwards, so you are in a hand plank position. Jump your legs back in, knees to your chest, so you return to your crouch position. Explode up into the air in a jump, landing back in your starting position. Repeat this move for the full minute.

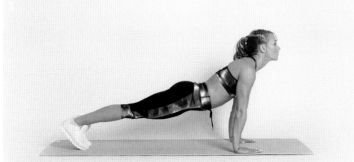

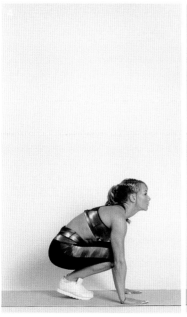

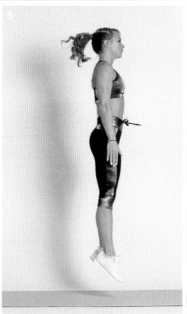

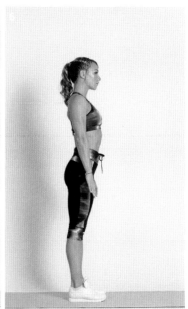

3 SIT UPS
x 1 minute

You will need a mat or a soft surface for this move. If you have never done ab exercises before, or you know you have a weak core, feel free to slide your feet under something to provide resistance – this will aid the sitting up movement. Lie flat on your back, keep your knees bent, with your legs and feet together. Sit up and gently lower yourself back down again. Repeat this movement for 1 minute.

Feel free to slide your feet under a secure surface to help perform Sit Ups – I do!

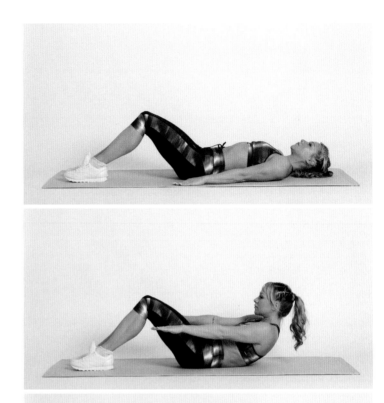

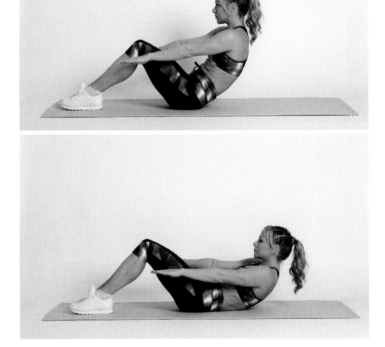

4 MOUNTAIN CLIMBERS x 1 minute

Lie on your front, feet hip-width apart, toes facing towards the floor. Place your hands by the sides of your chest, palms facing the floor. Push yourself up by your hands and feet. Bring one knee up to your chest and then back to the starting position. As you do this, switch legs, so you are essentially performing High Knees (see page 108) in a horizontal position. Continue for the full minute.

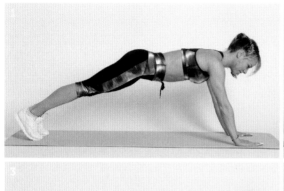
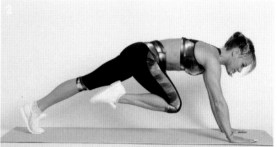
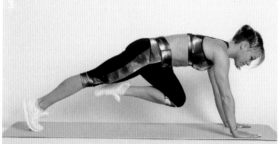
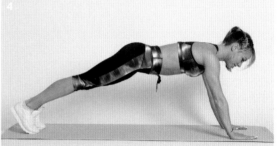

REST x 1 minute

**Repeat exercises 1–4
followed by a rest**
x 8 times
Total: 40 minutes

Cool down (see pages 43–54)

Tuesday's Diet:
High Fat, Low Carb

Build your own meals using **only** proteins, fats and non-starchy vegetables – see page 28 for explanation and portion sizes. For recipe ideas on what to have for breakfast, see pages 134–49, choose 2 snacks from the list on page 36 and for recipe ideas on what to have for lunch and dinner, see pages 168–83.

WARM UP
(see pages
43–54)

EXERCISES 1–4
back to back
and then rest
for 1 minute
Total: 5 minutes

REPEAT
exercises 1–4
followed by a rest
x 8 times
Total: 40 minutes

COOL DOWN
(see pages
43–54)

1 ELBOWS TO HAND PLANK
x 1 minute

You may need a mat or cushion for your elbows during this exercise. Lie on your front with your feet hip-width apart, resting your toes against the top of the mat. Rest on your elbows and keep your forearms flat against the mat. Keep your arms tucked in tight beside you. Pushing against your toes and forearms, raise your upper body into the air, one arm at a time, to rest on your hands, so you form an elevated plank. DO NOT allow your spine to curve, either concavely or convexly. You need a straight back, just like a plank. Come back down to rest on your forearms and then push back up onto your hands. Repeat this movement for 1 minute.

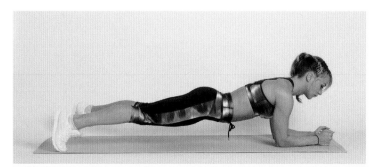

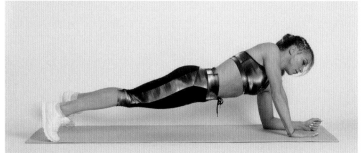

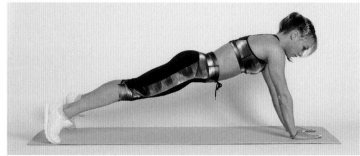

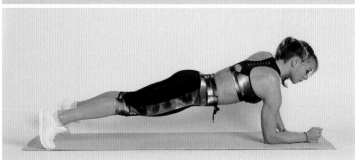

2 STAR JUMPS x 1 minute

Stand up straight with your feet together and your arms down at your sides. Jump your feet outwards (laterally) and, as you do so, bring your arms out and up over your head. Jump back into your starting position and repeat this move for 1 minute. This should be a controlled, fast-pace move.

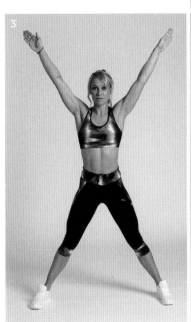
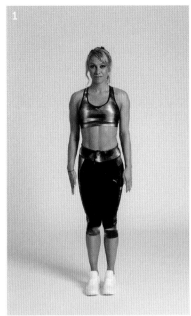
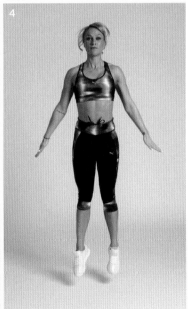
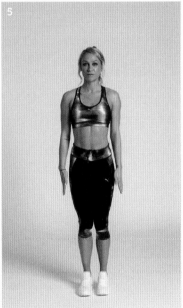
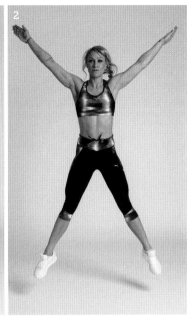

3 TRICEP DIPS
x 1 minute

You will need a chair, a step, a bench, or any slightly raised surface for this movement. Stand facing away from the chair. Place your palms down on to the chair and slowly lower your body down by bending at the elbows. Place your legs out in front of you and cross your ankles. Straighten your arms to raise yourself back up into your starting position. Repeat this move for 1 minute. Remember to keep your elbows in tight – they shouldn't be bowing outwards.

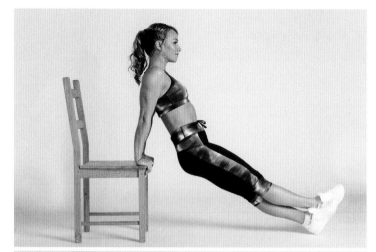

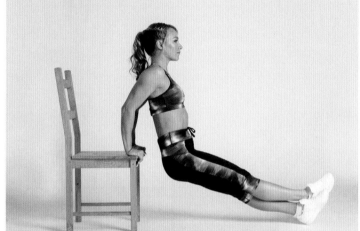

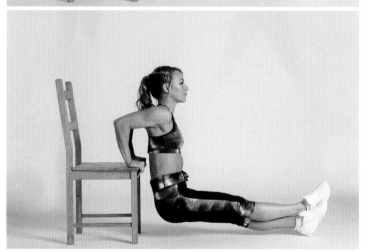

2 MOUNTAIN CLIMBERS x 1 minute

Lie on your front, feet hip-width apart, toes facing towards the floor. Place your hands by the sides of your chest, palms facing the floor. Push yourself up by your hands and feet. Bring one knee up to your chest and then back to the starting position. As you do this, switch legs, so you are essentially performing High Knees (see page 108) in a horizontal position. Continue for the full minute.

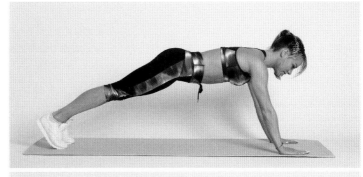

REST x 1 minute

Repeat exercises 1–4 followed by a rest
x 8 times
Total: 40 minutes

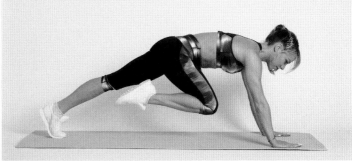

Cool down
(see pages 43–54)

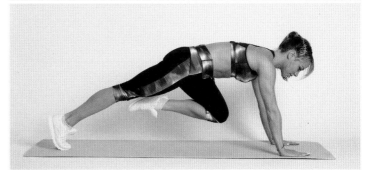

Wednesday's Diet:
High Fat, Low Carb

Build your own meals using **only** proteins, fats and non-starchy vegetables – see page 28 for explanation and portion sizes. For recipe ideas on what to have for breakfast, see pages 134–49, choose 2 snacks from the list on page 36 and for recipe ideas on what to have for lunch and dinner, see pages 168–83.

WARM UP (see pages 43–54)

EXERCISES 1–4 back to back and then rest for 1 minute
Total: 5 minutes

REPEAT exercises 1–4 followed by a rest x 8 times
Total: 40 minutes

COOL DOWN (see pages 43–54)

1 MOUNTAIN CLIMBERS x 1 minute

Lie on your front, feet hip-width apart, toes facing towards the floor. Place your hands by the sides of your chest, palms facing the floor. Push yourself up by your hands and feet. Bring one knee up to your chest and then back to the starting position. As you do this, switch legs, so you are essentially performing High Knees (see page 108) in a horizontal position. Continue for the full minute.

You're in week 4 now – PUSH!

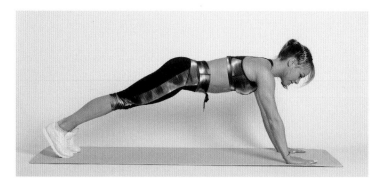

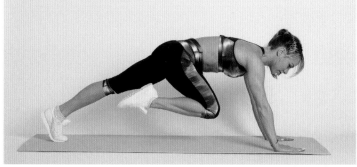

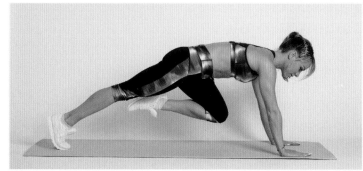

2 WALK OUT PUSH UPS
x 1 minute

Stand up straight with your feet hip-width apart. Allowing your knees to bend slightly, come down and forward out in front of yourself, allowing your hands to touch the floor, palms flat, and place them shoulder-width apart. Crawl outwards until you are fully extended in a horizontal position. Keeping your back straight and bending only at the elbows, perform a push up. Crawl back on yourself until you can stand upright again. Repeat this move for 1 minute.

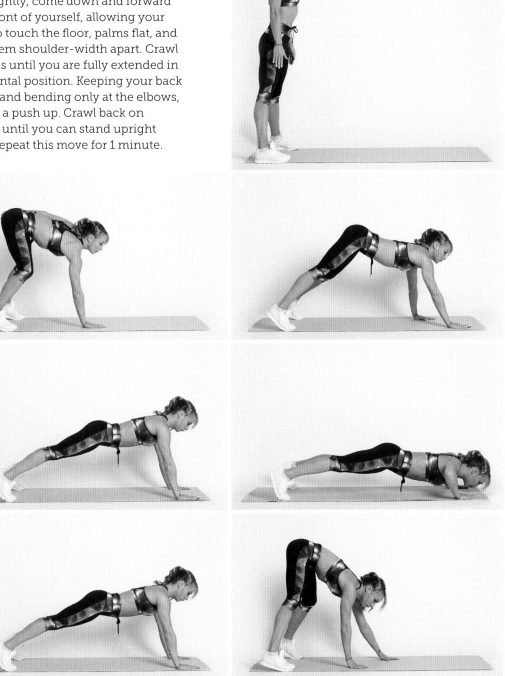

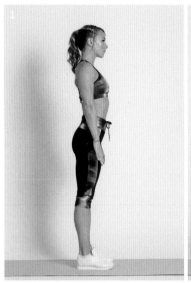

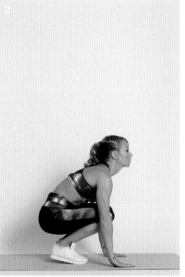

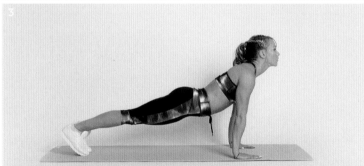

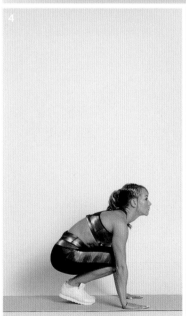

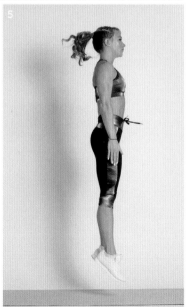

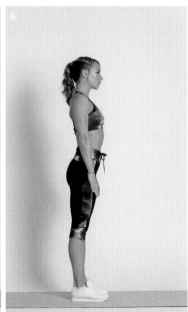

3 BURPEES
x 1 minute

Stand up straight with your feet together and your arms down by your sides. Come down into a crouch (think like a frog) and place your palms flat on the ground in front of you. Put your body weight on your hands and jump your legs backwards, so you are in a hand plank position. Jump your legs back in, knees to your chest, so you return to your crouch position. Explode up into the air in a jump, landing back in your starting position. Repeat this move for the full minute.

4 SQUAT JUMPS x 1 minute

Stand up straight with your feet hip-width apart. Extend your arms directly out in front of you and place one hand on top of the other – alternatively, place your hands on your hips. Keeping your back straight, lower yourself down into a deep squat by bending your knees. Instead of standing back up again from the squat, gently jump back into a standing position. The jump should be so gentle that you can maintain your form from the very start of the exercise to the next repetition. It should also be so gentle that you only come off the floor a little. Bear in mind that big dynamic jumps can damage your joints, so keep it gentle. Repeat this move for 1 minute.

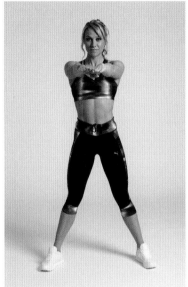 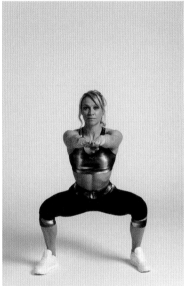 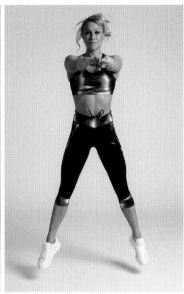

REST x 1 minute

Repeat exercises 1–4 followed by a rest
x 8 times
Total: 40 minutes

Cool down (see pages 43–54)

Thursday's Diet:
High Fat, Low Carb

Build your own meals using **only** proteins, fats and non-starchy vegetables – see page 28 for explanation and portion sizes. For recipe ideas on what to have for breakfast, see pages 134–49, choose 2 snacks from the list on page 36 and for recipe ideas on what to have for lunch and dinner, see pages 168–83.

WEEK 4 FRIDAY

WARM UP (see pages 43–54)

Perform any circuit of your choice **Exercises 1–4 back to back and then rest for 1 minute** Total: 5 minutes

REPEAT exercises 1–4 followed by a rest x 8 times Total: 40 minutes

COOL DOWN (see pages 43–54)

Friday's Diet: High Fat, Low Carb

Build your meals using **only** proteins, fats and non-starchy vegetables – see page 28 for explanation and portion sizes. For recipe ideas on what to have for breakfast, see pages 134–49, choose 2 snacks from the list on page 36 and for recipe ideas on what to have for lunch and dinner, see pages 168–83.

WEEK 4 SATURDAY

WARM UP (see pages 43–54)

Perform any circuit of your choice **Exercises 1–4 back to back and then rest for 1 minute** Total: 5 minutes

REPEAT exercises 1–4 followed by a rest x 8 times Total: 40 minutes

COOL DOWN (see pages 43–54)

Saturday's Diet: High Carb, Low Fat

Build your meals using **only** proteins, non-starchy vegetables and carbs – see page 28 for explanation and portion sizes. For recipe ideas on what to have for breakfast, see pages 152–64, choose 2 snacks from the list on page 36 and for recipe ideas on what to have for lunch and dinner, see pages 186–99.

WEEK 4 SUNDAY

Rest day

Sunday's Diet: High Fat, Low Carb

Build your meals using **only** proteins, fats and non-starchy vegetables – see page 28 for explanation and portion sizes. For recipe ideas on what to have for breakfast, see pages 134–49, choose 2 snacks from the list on page 36 and for recipe ideas on what to have for lunch and dinner, see pages 168–83.

Congratulations!
You have now completed
The 4-Week Body Blitz!
Exercising hard 5–6 days a week is a huge effort and a huge accomplishment and you should feel incredibly proud of yourself!
WELL DONE!

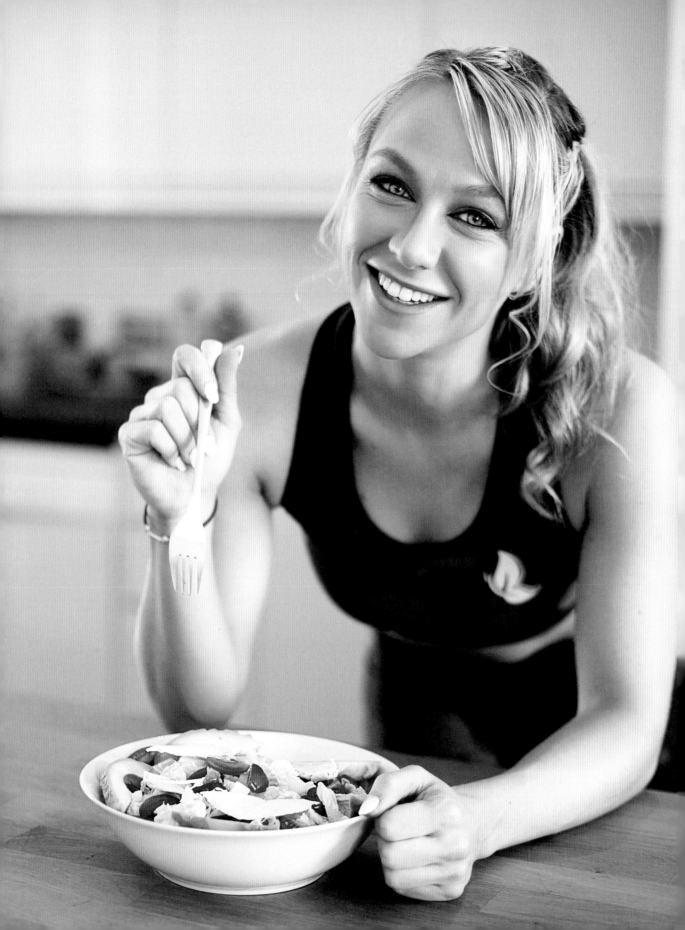

RECIPES

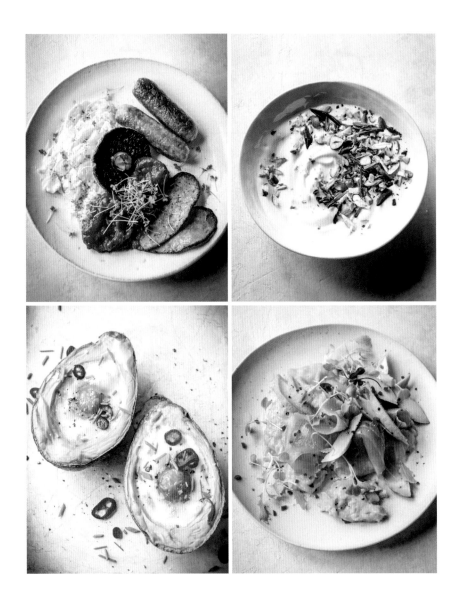

HIGH FAT
BREAKFASTS
LOW CARB

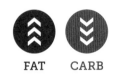

FAT   CARB

Mexican Scrambled Eggs

I like to add a dash of Tabasco when I'm scrambling the eggs to give the dish a bit of a kick, and I'll top it with fresh herbs to add colour and freshness – parsley or coriander work well.

SERVES 1

Quantities for Women
1 level tsp butter
1 heaped tbsp diced red
    onion
½ jalapeño pepper, sliced
3 whole eggs
½ avocado, peeled and diced
½ tomato, diced
seasoning, to taste

Quantities for Men
1 heaped tsp butter
2 level tbsp diced red onion
1 jalapeño pepper, sliced
4–5 whole eggs
½–1 avocado, peeled
    and diced
½–1 tomato, diced
seasoning, to taste

1 Melt the butter in a frying pan over a medium heat.

2 Add the onion and jalapeño and allow to soften for 2–3 minutes.

3 Crack the eggs into the pan and scramble with the other ingredients, using a whisk or spatula, until the preferred consistency is reached.

4 Remove from the pan and top with the diced avocado and tomato, season to taste and serve.

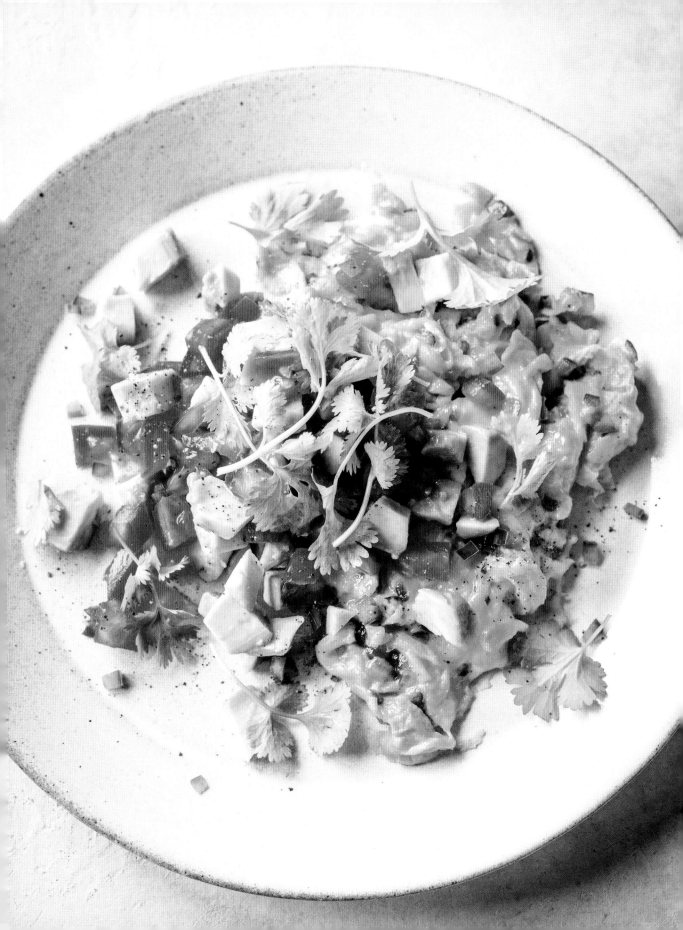

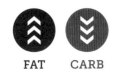

FAT   CARB

Breakfast Shake

I add ice cubes before whizzing – I use three, but you could add more or less. Look out for nut butters without any added oils or sugar – these are 'clean' nut butters.

MAKES 1 PINT

Quantities for Women
1 scoop whey protein powder (typically 25–35g)
1 level tbsp any clean nut butter (peanut / almond / cashew)
1 heaped tbsp full-fat Greek yoghurt
400ml unsweetened almond milk

Quantities for Men
1½ scoops whey protein powder (typically 40–50g)
1 heaped tbsp any clean nut butter (peanut / almond / cashew)
2 level tbsp full-fat Greek yoghurt
600ml unsweetened almond milk

1 Place all the ingredients in a blender and whizz to your preferred consistency.

2 Pour into a large glass and serve.

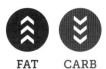

FAT   CARB

Steak and Eggs

When I'm particularly hungry, this is what I'll have for breakfast!

SERVES 1

Quantities for Women

1 small steak (typically
    150–200g), any cut
2 whole eggs
seasoning, to taste

Quantities for Men

1 large steak (typically
    225–300g), any cut
3 whole eggs
seasoning, to taste

1 Allow the steak to sit and come up to room temperature before cooking.

2 Place a frying pan over a high heat and leave it to become smoking hot.

3 Place the steak in the pan, season and fry for 1 minute. Turn and fry on the other side for a further minute, or until cooked to your preference.

4 Remove the steak from the pan and place on a plate to rest.

5 Return the pan to the heat and crack in the eggs. Scramble with a whisk, or fry them, depending on your preference.

6 Remove the eggs on to the plate with the steak, season to taste and serve.

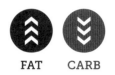

FAT   CARB

Greek Yoghurt Bowl

My favourite nuts to use are almonds because they go so well
with the chocolate.

SERVES 1

Quantities for Women
1 small pot full-fat Greek
　yoghurt (typically 170g)
1 small handful any nuts,
　roughly chopped
1 large square 90% dark
　chocolate (typically 20g),
　grated

Quantities for Men
1½ small pots full-fat Greek
　yoghurt (typically 255g)
1 large handful any nuts,
　roughly chopped
1½ large squares 90% dark
　chocolate (typically 45g),
　grated

1 Combine the yoghurt and nuts together
in a bowl and mix well.

2 Sprinkle over the dark chocolate and serve.

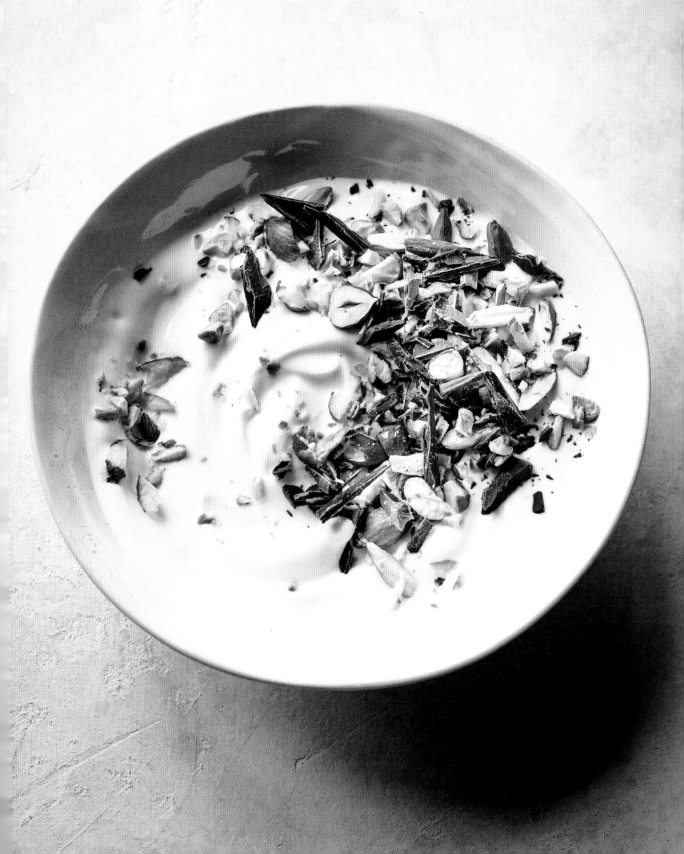

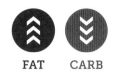

FAT **CARB**

Avocado, Smoked Salmon and Scrambled Eggs

Try seasoning the scrambled eggs with plenty of black pepper and a pinch of sea salt and then sprinkling rocket over the finished dish before eating.

SERVES 1

Quantities for Women

1 level tsp butter
3 whole eggs
50g smoked salmon, torn into strips
½ small avocado, peeled and sliced
seasoning, to taste

Quantities for Men

1 heaped tsp butter
4–5 whole eggs
75g smoked salmon, torn into strips
1 small or ½ large avocado, peeled and sliced
seasoning, to taste

1 Melt the butter in a frying pan over a medium heat.

2 Crack in the eggs and scramble, using a whisk or spatula.

3 Once the eggs are almost at your preferred consistency, carefully tip onto a plate.

4 Top with the salmon and sliced avocado, season to taste and serve.

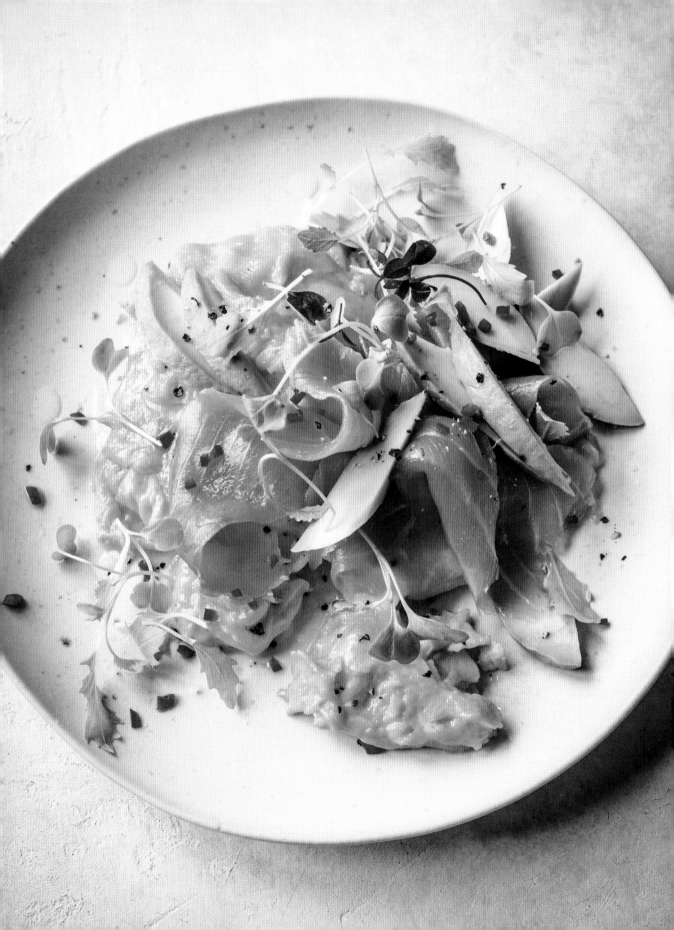

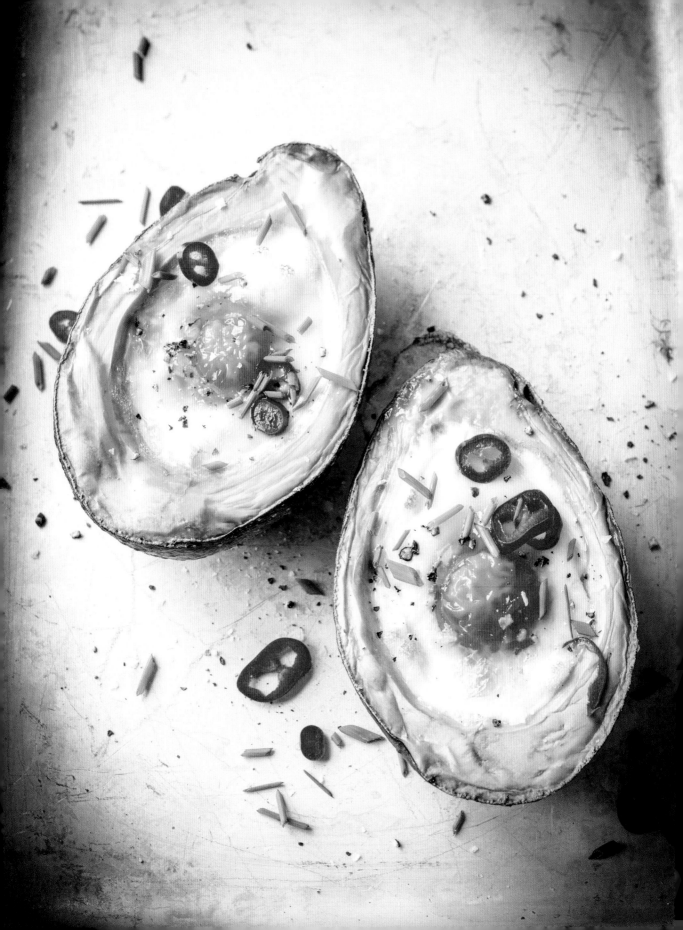

FAT   CARB

Avocado Eggs

Garnish with fresh chilli and a squeeze of lime, or season with salt and pepper and a sprinkling of fresh dill or chopped chives.

MAKES 2

Quantities for Women
1 avocado, halved
    and destoned
2 whole eggs
seasoning, to taste

Quantities for Men
1½ avocados, halved
    and destoned
3 whole eggs
seasoning, to taste

1 Preheat the oven to 220°C.

2 Place the avocado halves in an oven dish cut side upwards and crack an egg into the circular space left by the stone in each avocado half.

3 Season with salt and pepper and then bake in the oven for 15–20 minutes.

4 Remove from the oven and serve.

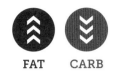

FAT **CARB**

Nut Butter Protein Pancakes

Make sure the batter is thick and BE PATIENT! Protein pancakes can take a few minutes before they are ready to be flipped.

MAKES 2–3

Quantities for Women

1 scoop whey protein powder (typically 25–35g)

1 whole egg

200ml unsweetened almond milk

1 level tsp coconut oil

1 level tbsp any clean nut butter (peanut / almond / cashew)

Quantities for Men

1½ scoops whey protein powder (typically 40–55g)

2 whole eggs

300ml unsweetened almond milk

1 heaped tsp coconut oil

1 heaped tbsp any clean nut butter (peanut / almond / cashew)

1 Combine the protein powder, egg and almond milk in a jug and mix together well with a fork.

2 Melt the coconut oil in a frying pan over a medium heat.

3 Pour some batter into the centre of the pan and cook for 1–2 minutes. Turn the pancake over and cook for a further minute, or until both sides are golden brown.

4 Remove from the pan onto a plate and keep warm while you continue to cook the remaining pancakes.

5 Drizzle the pancakes with the nut butter and serve.

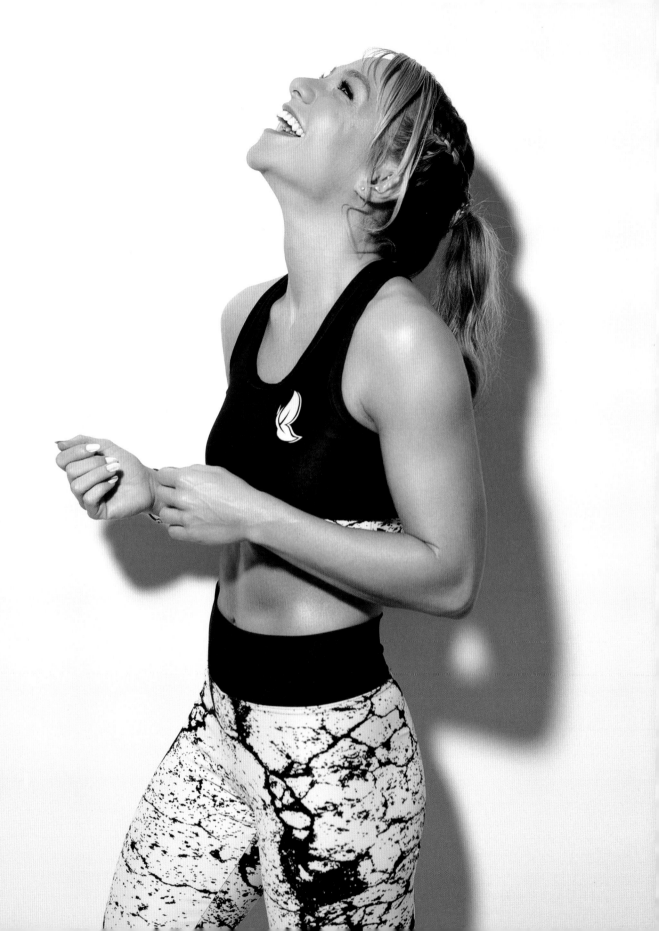

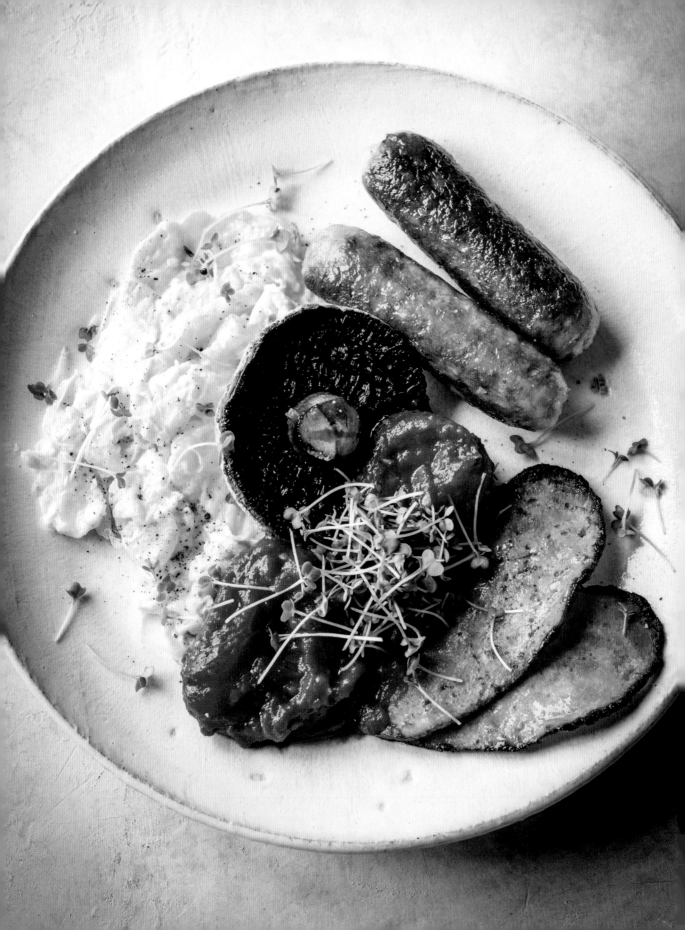

FAT CARB

English Breakfast

You don't need to miss out on your weekend fry up if you tweak a few ingredients here and there.

SERVES 1

Quantities for Women
2 chicken sausages
½ x 400g tin peeled
 plum tomatoes
1 Portobello mushroom
2 slices turkey bacon
2 whole eggs
seasoning, to taste

Quantities for Men
3 chicken sausages
¾ x 400g tin peeled
 plum tomatoes
1½ Portobello mushrooms
3 slices turkey bacon
3 whole eggs
seasoning, to taste

1 Preheat the grill to medium-high.

2 Pierce the chicken sausages with a fork and grill for 15 minutes, turning occasionally.

3 Meanwhile, place the peeled plum tomatoes in a pan over a medium heat and leave to simmer for 5–10 minutes. Season to taste.

4 While the tomatoes are bubbling, add the Portobello mushroom and turkey rashers to the grill tray and cook for 3–4 minutes on each side.

5 Finally, cook the eggs in your preferred way, season to taste and serve with the sausages, tomatoes, mushroom and turkey rashers.

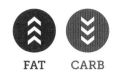

FAT **CARB**

Egg Stacks

This is my favourite mid-week breakfast, and once you try it you'll never look back. Just as delicious as eggs Benedict with a fraction of the calories.

MAKES 2

Quantities for Women
2 Portobello mushrooms
2 slices turkey bacon
1 level tsp butter
2 whole eggs
½ avocado, peeled and sliced thinly
seasoning, to taste

Quantities for Men
3 Portobello mushrooms
3 slices turkey bacon
1 heaped tsp butter
3 whole eggs
1 small or ½ large avocado, peeled and sliced thinly
seasoning, to taste

1 Preheat the grill to medium-high.

2 Place the Portobello mushrooms and turkey rashers under the grill and cook for 3–4 minutes on each side.

3 Meanwhile, melt the butter in a frying pan over a medium heat.

4 Crack in the eggs and fry until they are cooked to your preference.

5 Place the mushrooms side by side on a plate and then stack the remaining ingredients on top of each mushroom in the following order: first the avocado slices, then an egg and finally top each one with a turkey rasher.

6 Season to taste and serve.

FAT   CARB

Overnight Chia Bowl

If you would prefer to have this warm on a cold morning, you can pop it in the microwave for 1–2 minutes, or warm through in a pan over a medium heat – just make sure you heat it before adding the nuts, cinnamon and agave syrup.

SERVES 1

Quantities for Women

4 level tbsp chia seeds

100ml unsweetened almond milk (enough to just about cover the seeds)

1 level tbsp chopped / crushed almonds

¼ tsp ground cinnamon

1 tsp agave syrup

Quantities for Men

6 level tbsp chia seeds

150ml unsweetened almond milk (enough to just about cover the seeds)

1 heaped tbsp chopped / crushed almonds

½ tsp ground cinnamon

1½ tsp agave syrup

1 Mix the seeds and almond milk in a bowl and leave in the fridge overnight.

2 When ready to serve, stir in the nuts, sprinkle with the cinnamon and drizzle with the agave syrup.

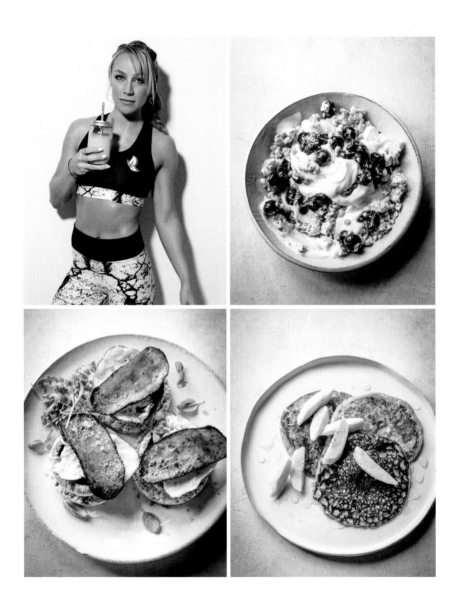

HIGH CARB
BREAKFASTS
LOW FAT

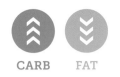

CARB   FAT

Proats

If you don't like bananas, you could grate
1 small apple over the oats instead.

SERVES 1

Quantities for Women
50g plain oats (typically 2
 sachets or 2 heaped tbsp)
1 scoop whey protein powder
 (typically 25–35g)
boiling water
1 small or ½ large banana,
 sliced

Quantities for Men
75g plain oats (typically 3
 sachets or 3 heaped tbsp)
1½ scoops whey protein
 powder (typically 40–55g)
boiling water
2 small or 1 large banana,
 sliced

1 Mix the oats and protein powder together in a bowl. Add small dashes of boiling water from the kettle until the desired consistency has been reached.

2 Top with the banana and serve.

CARB FAT

Rice Cake Krispies

Instead of cinnamon, you could flavour
the Krispies with ground ginger.

SERVES 1

Quantities for Women
5 plain rice cakes
1 scoop whey protein powder
    (typically 25–35g)
400ml water
½ tsp ground cinnamon

Quantities for Men
8 plain rice cakes
1½ scoops whey protein
    powder (typically 40–55g)
600ml water
1 tsp ground cinnamon

1 Crush the rice cakes into a bowl with your
hands.

2 Combine the protein powder with the water
in a jug and mix well.

3 Pour the protein water over the crushed rice
cakes, sprinkle with the cinnamon and serve.

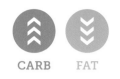

CARB FAT

Breakfast Smoothie

You can add ice cubes before whizzing in the blender
if you want a different texture and temperature.

MAKES 1 PINT

Quantities for Women

1 scoop whey protein powder
  (typically 25–35g)
25g plain oats (typically
  1 sachet or 1 heaped tbsp)
1 heaped tbsp 0% fat Greek
  yoghurt
1 small or ½ large banana
450ml unsweetened
  almond milk

Quantities for Men

1½ scoops whey protein
  powder (typically 40–55g)
40g plain oats (typically
  1½ sachets or 2 tbsp)
2 level tbsp 0% fat Greek
  yoghurt
2 small or 1 large banana
675ml unsweetened
  almond milk

1 Place all the ingredients in a blender
and whizz.

2 Pour into a large glass and serve.

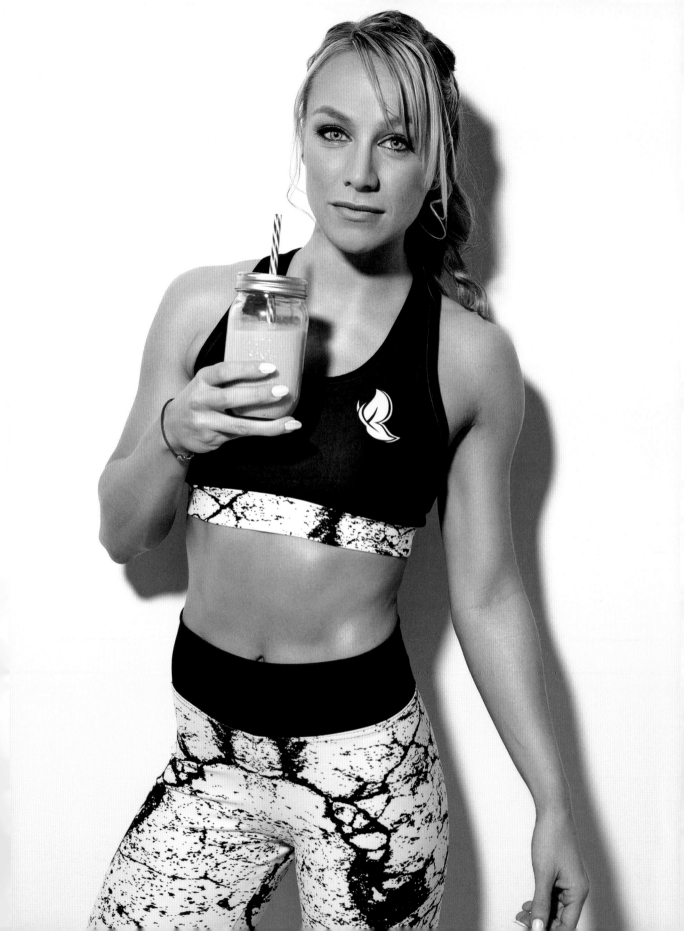

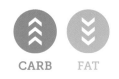

CARB   FAT

Overnight Oats

Like with other recipes, you can always replace the
banana with an apple, which would go especially
well with the cinnamon.

SERVES 1

Quantities for Women
50g plain oats (typically 2
    sachets or 2 heaped tbsp)
200ml unsweetened
    almond milk
1 heaped tbsp 0% fat
    Greek yoghurt
1 large banana, peeled and
    chopped into small chunks
½ tsp ground cinnamon

Quantities for Men
75g plain oats (typically 3
    sachets or 3 heaped tbsp)
300ml unsweetened almond
    milk
2 level tbsp 0% fat
    Greek yoghurt
1½ large bananas, peeled and
    chopped into small chunks
1 tsp ground cinnamon

1 Mix all the ingredients together in a bowl.

2 Cover with cling film and leave in the fridge
overnight (or for a minimum of 4 hours).

3 Remove from the fridge and serve.

CARB   FAT

English Breakfast with American Spuds

Try tossing the potato cubes in salt, pepper and a pinch of mustard powder before roasting, and chop fresh parsley to garnish the finished dish.

SERVES 1

Quantities for Women

1 small potato (typically 150–200g), washed and chopped into small cubes
2 chicken sausages
½ x 400g tin peeled plum tomatoes
1 Portobello mushroom
2 slices turkey bacon
2 large egg whites
seasoning, to taste

Quantities for Men

1 large potato (typically 225–300g), washed and chopped into small cubes
3 chicken sausages
¾ x 400g tin peeled plum tomatoes
1½ Portobello mushrooms
3 slices turkey bacon
3 large egg whites
seasoning, to taste

1 Preheat the oven to 220°C.

2 Place the potato on a baking tray and season well.

3 Bake in the oven for 20 minutes.

4 Meanwhile, preheat the grill to medium-high.

5 Pierce the chicken sausages with a fork and cook under the grill for 15 minutes, turning occasionally.

6 Place the tomatoes in a small pan over a medium heat, season to taste and allow to simmer for 5–10 minutes.

7 Add the Portobello mushroom and turkey rashers to the tray under the grill and allow both to cook for 3–4 minutes on each side.

8 Finally, cook the egg whites in your preferred way and season to taste.

9 Serve the egg whites with the potatoes, sausages, tomatoes, mushroom and turkey rashers.

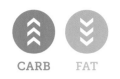

CARB   FAT

Greek Mess

If you don't have any blueberries, try another berry.
I like using strawberries, as they are so sweet!

SERVES 1

Quantities for Women
1 small pot 0% fat Greek
   yoghurt (typically 170g)
5 plain rice cakes
1 small handful blueberries
1 level tsp agave syrup

Quantities for Men
1½ small pots 0% fat Greek
   yoghurt (typically 250g)
8 plain rice cakes
1½ small handfuls
   blueberries
1 heaped tsp agave syrup

1 Spoon the yoghurt into a serving bowl.

2 Using your hands, crush the rice cakes over the yoghurt.

3 Bruise the blueberries gently so that they release a bit of their juice as you add them to the bowl.

4 Mix together well, drizzle with the agave syrup and serve.

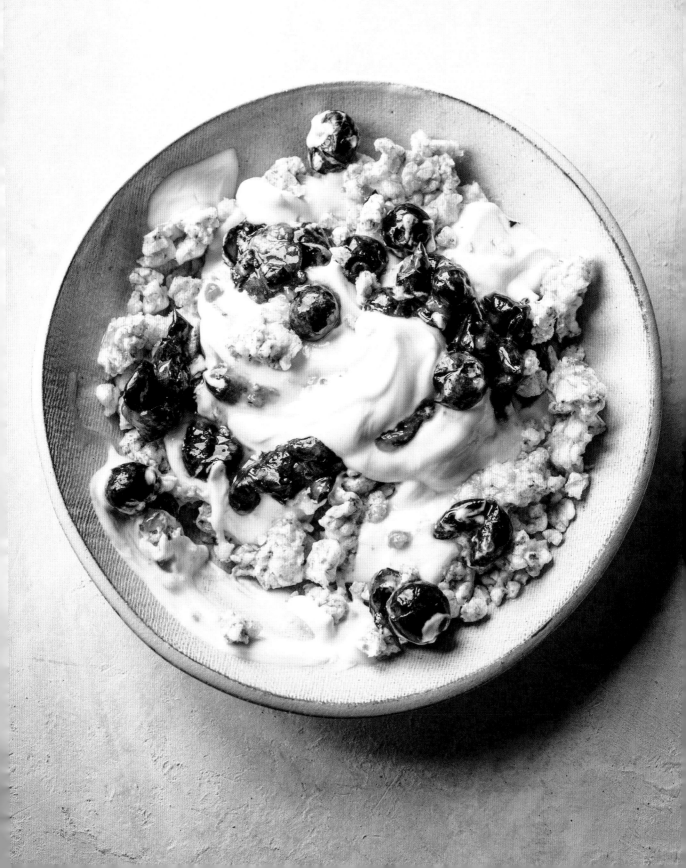

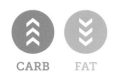

CARB FAT

Proat Pancakes

These pancakes are my favourite high carb
and low fat breakfast.

MAKES 3

Quantities for Women
1 large banana
1 scoop whey protein powder
    (typically 25–35g)
25g plain oats (typically 1
    sachet or 1 heaped tbsp)
200ml unsweetened almond
    milk
a light drizzle of agave syrup

Quantities for Men
1½ large bananas
1½ scoops whey protein
    powder (typically 40–55g)
40g plain oats (typically 1½
    sachets or 2 tbsp)
300ml unsweetened
    almond milk
a light drizzle of agave syrup

1 Cut the banana in two and slice one half into
bitesize pieces. Mash the other half with a fork.

2 Place the mashed banana, protein powder,
oats and almond milk in a large jug and whisk
everything together well.

3 Place a non-stick pan over a high heat and
leave it to become smoking hot.

4 Pour some batter into the centre of the pan
and cook until both sides are golden brown.

5 Remove the pancake to a plate and keep
warm while you cook the remaining batter.

6 When all the pancakes have been cooked,
serve topped with the sliced banana and
drizzled lightly with agave syrup.

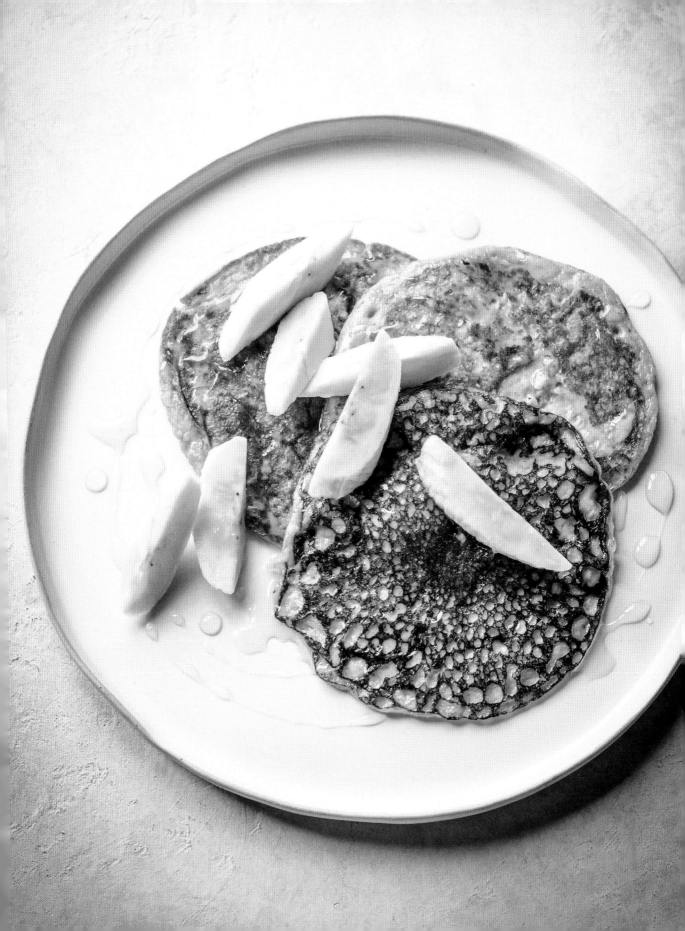

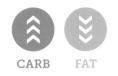

CARB FAT

Rancheros Cakes

I like to add Tabasco to the finished dish and scatter
fresh herbs over the cakes, too.

MAKES 4

Quantities for Women
1 heaped tbsp diced
    red onion
½ jalapeño pepper, diced
6 large egg whites
4 plain rice cakes
½ tomato, diced
seasoning, to taste

Quantities for Men
2 tbsp diced red onion
1 jalapeño pepper, diced
9 large egg whites
6 plain rice cakes
1 tomato, diced
seasoning, to taste

1 Place a non-stick frying pan over a high heat
and leave it to get smoking hot.

2 Add the diced onion and jalapeño and allow
to cook for 2–3 minutes.

3 Add the egg whites to the pan and scramble
the ingredients together using a whisk or
spatula.

4 Meanwhile, place the rice cakes on a serving
plate.

5 Once the eggs are your preferred consistency,
remove from the pan and place carefully on top
of the rice cakes.

6 Garnish each cake with some diced tomato,
season to taste and serve.

CARB   FAT

Lean Steak, Whites and Spuds

Sprinkle the potatoes with paprika before roasting in the oven and season the steak with salt and pepper. I garnish the eggs with freshly chopped parsley, too.

SERVES 1

Quantities for Women

1 small lean steak (typically 150–200g), any cut

1 small potato (typically 150–200g), washed and diced (no need to peel)

3 large egg whites

seasoning, to taste

Quantities for Men

1 large lean steak (typically 225–300g), any cut

1 large potato (typically 225–300g), washed and diced (no need to peel)

5 large egg whites

seasoning, to taste

1 Preheat the oven to 220°C.

2 Allow the steak to sit and come up to room temperature before cooking.

3 Place the potato on a baking tray and season well.

4 Cook the potato in the oven for 20 minutes.

5 Place a frying pan over a high heat and leave it to become smoking hot.

6 Add the steak to the pan, season and sear on each side for 1 minute, or until cooked to your preference.

7 Remove from the pan and place on a plate to rest.

8 Meanwhile, add the egg whites to the pan, turn the heat down to medium and scramble with a whisk or spatula until they are your preferred consistency.

9 Season the eggs to taste and serve alongside the steak and potatoes.

HIGH CARB, LOW FAT BREAKFASTS **163**

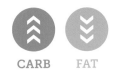

CARB   FAT

Breakfast Cakes

This is a great flavour combination.

MAKES 3

Quantities for Women
3 Portobello mushrooms
3 slices turkey bacon
3 large egg whites
3 plain rice cakes
seasoning, to taste

Quantities for Men
5 Portobello mushrooms
5 slices turkey bacon
5 large egg whites
5 plain rice cakes
seasoning, to taste

1 Preheat the grill to medium-high.

2 Place the Portobello mushrooms and turkey rashers under the grill and cook for 3–4 minutes on each side.

3 Meanwhile, fry the egg whites in a non-stick pan over a high heat to your preferred consistency.

4 Place the rice cakes on a plate and top each one with a mushroom, then some egg white, and finally a turkey rasher.

5 Season to taste and serve.

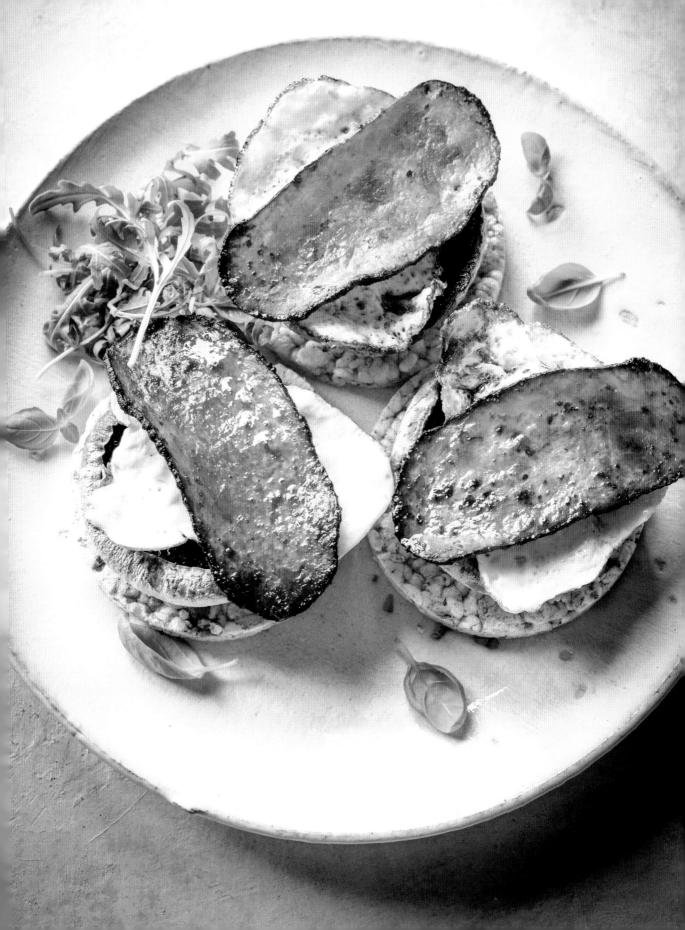

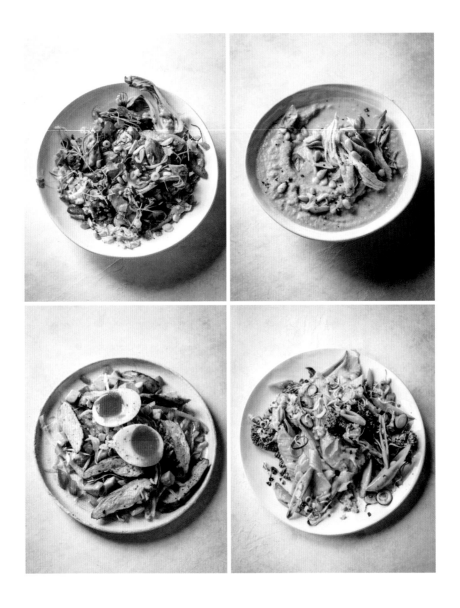

HIGH FAT
LUNCHES
AND
DINNERS
LOW CARB

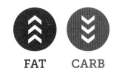

FAT CARB

Courgetti Bolognaise

I sometimes add dried herbs after I've browned the mince –
oregano is a particular favourite and a pinch is usually enough –
or I'll sprinkle a few dried chilli flakes over the bolognaise before
serving, if I fancy a bit of spice. If I have salad in the fridge,
I'll garnish the courgetti with a few leaves of rocket to give
it a lovely peppery flavour.

SERVES 1

Quantities for Women
1 large courgette
small dash olive oil
½ small onion, peeled
  and diced
½ tsp chopped garlic
125g 5% fat beef mince
½ x 400g tin chopped
  tomatoes
seasoning, to taste

Quantities for Men
1½ large courgettes
small dash olive oil
½ large onion, peeled
  and diced
1 tsp chopped garlic
185g 5% fat beef mince
¾ x 400g tin chopped
  tomatoes
seasoning, to taste

1 Grate the courgette into long strands
(vertically down the largest slicing option
on a cheese grater will do the trick – or
you could use a spiraliser).

2 Put the oil into a pan over a medium heat.

3 Add the onion and garlic and allow to soften
for 2–3 minutes.

4 Add the mince and cook for 2–3 minutes,
or until brown.

5 Pour in the chopped tomatoes and stir
well. Season to taste and leave to simmer
for 5–10 minutes.

6 Stir in the grated courgette and allow to
simmer for a further 5–10 minutes.

7 Remove from the heat, check the seasoning
and serve.

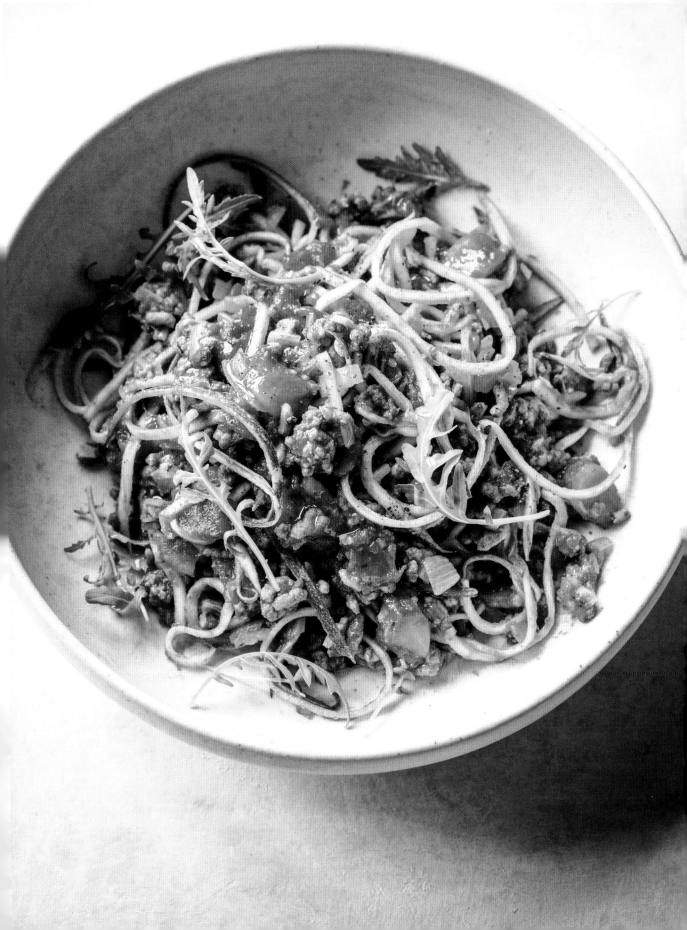

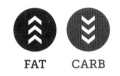

FAT   CARB

Chilli Con Carne and Cauliflower Rice

Add chilli powder, as well as the fresh chillies,
if you like it spicy. Cauliflower rice is a great substitute
for rice on a low carb day.

SERVES 1

Quantities for Women
½ small cauliflower head
   (typically 125g)
dash olive oil
small onion, peeled
   and chopped
½ tsp chopped garlic
125g 5% beef mince
1–2 chillies, chopped
½ x 400g tin chopped
   tomatoes
seasoning, to taste

Quantities for Men
1 large cauliflower head
   (typically 200g)
dash olive oil
½ large onion, peeled
   and chopped
1 tsp chopped garlic
185g 5% beef mince
1–2 chillies, chopped
¾ x 400g tin chopped
   tomatoes
seasoning, to taste

1 Break the cauliflower into florets and place
in a food processor and whizz, or grate with
a cheese grater until riced. Season to taste.

2 Place the oil in a pan over a medium heat.

3 Add the onion and garlic and leave to soften
for 2–3 minutes.

4 Add the mince to the pan and cook for
2–3 minutes until brown.

5 Add the chillies and tomatoes to the pan
and stir well. Season to taste and leave to
simmer for 5–10 minutes.

6 Meanwhile, warm the cauliflower in a
microwave for 1–2 minutes.

7 Place the cauliflower on a large plate and
pour over the chilli. Check the seasoning
and serve.

FAT   CARB

Chicken Sausage and Broccoli Mash

It may seem strange to cook the broccoli this long but you need it to be really soft in order to mash it.

SERVES 1

Quantities for Women

4 chicken sausages

1 small broccoli head (typically 200g), broken into florets

1 level tbsp salted butter

seasoning, to taste

Quantities for Men

6 chicken sausages

1 large broccoli head (typically 300g), broken into florets

1 heaped tbsp salted butter

seasoning, to taste

1 Preheat the grill to medium-high.

2 Pierce the chicken sausages with a fork and place under the grill for 15 minutes, turning occasionally.

3 Bring a large pan of salted water to the boil, add the broccoli and cook for 20 minutes (you need to cook it to within an inch of its life – the broccoli has to be very soft).

4 Drain the broccoli, tip back into the pan and add the butter. Mash well and season to taste.

5 Scoop the mash into a serving bowl, top with the sausages and serve.

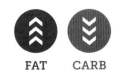

FAT   **CARB**

Peanut Butter Chicken Stir-Fry

Garnish this stir-fry with sprigs of fresh coriander and some sliced chilli and spring onion.

SERVES 1

Quantities for Women

1 chicken breast (typically 120g), cut into chunks
2 tbsp soy sauce
150g mixed vegetables, finely sliced or ½ pack ready-prepared stir-fry veg
1 level tbsp crunchy clean peanut butter
1 level tbsp salted peanuts
seasoning, to taste

Quantities for Men

1½ chicken breasts (typically 180g), diced
3 tbsp soy sauce
225g mixed vegetables, finely sliced or 1 pack ready-prepared stir-fry veg
1 heaped tbsp crunchy peanut butter
1 heaped tbsp salted peanuts
seasoning, to taste

1 Place the chicken in a bowl and mix with the soy sauce.

2 Place a non-stick pan over a medium heat and add the chicken and soy. Stir-fry for 4–5 minutes, or until lightly browned.

3 Add the veg and stir-fry for 3–4 minutes.

4 Remove the pan from the heat and stir in the peanut butter.

5 Tip into a serving bowl and sprinkle with the peanuts.

6 Season to taste and serve.

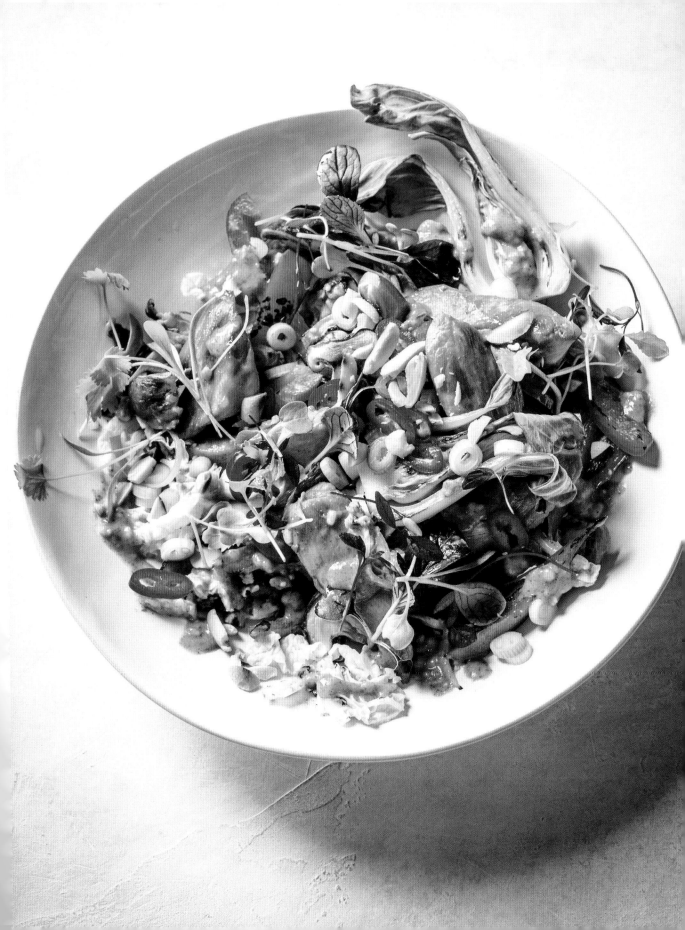

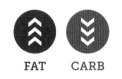

FAT   CARB

Chicken Napolitano Courgetti

Use fresh basil if you can and add it at the end,
instead of with the garlic.

SERVES 1

Quantities for Women

1 large courgette
1 chicken breast (typically
    120g), diced
1 tbsp olive oil
1 tsp chopped garlic
1 pinch dried basil
½ x 400g tin chopped
    tomatoes
seasoning, to taste

Quantities for Men

1½ large courgettes
1½ chicken breasts (typically
    180g), diced
4 tsp olive oil
1½ tsp chopped garlic
1 large pinch dried basil
¾ x 400g tin chopped
    tomatoes
seasoning, to taste

1 Grate the courgette into long strands
(vertically down the largest slicing option on
a cheese grater will do the trick – or you could
use a spiraliser).

2 Place a non-stick pan over a medium heat,
add the chicken and cook for 4–5 minutes,
or until brown.

3 Meanwhile, measure the olive oil into a
separate pan over a medium heat.

4 Add the garlic and basil and stir to coat
in the oil.

5 Stir in the chopped tinned tomatoes and
season to taste. Leave to simmer for 5 minutes.

6 Add the chicken and courgetti to the tomato
sauce and leave to simmer for a further
5 minutes.

7 Pour into a bowl, check the seasoning and
serve.

FAT CARB

Steak and Broccoli Mash

Sprinkle with plenty of freshly ground pepper
before serving.

SERVES 1

Quantities for Women

1 small steak (typically
    150–200g), any cut
1 small broccoli head
    (typically 200g), broken
    into florets
1 level tbsp salted butter
seasoning, to taste

Quantities for Men

1 large steak (typically
    225–300g), any cut
1 large broccoli head
    (typically 225g), broken
    into florets
1 heaped tbsp salted butter
seasoning, to taste

1 Allow the steak to sit and come up to
room temperature before cooking.

2 Bring a large pan of salted water to the
boil, add the broccoli and cook for 20 minutes
(you need to cook it to within an inch of its life
– the broccoli has to be very soft).

3 Drain the broccoli and tip back into the pan.
Season to taste, add the butter and mash well.

4 Meanwhile, place a frying pan over a high
heat and leave it to become smoking hot.

5 Season the steak then sear in the pan on
each side for 1 minute, or until cooked to
your preference.

6 Remove the steak and place on a plate to rest.

7 Check the seasoning of the broccoli and then
serve alongside the steak.

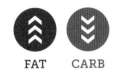

FAT   CARB

Mexican Cauli Rice Bowl

I like to add Tabasco, fresh chilli and a pinch of ground
paprika to the chicken when I marinate it.

SERVES 1

Quantities for Women
1 chicken breast
    (typically 120g)
juice of 1 lime
½ small cauliflower head
    (typically 125g)
½ small red onion,
    peeled and diced
1 small tomato, diced
1 jalapeño pepper, diced
½ avocado, peeled and diced
seasoning, to taste

Quantities for Men
1½ chicken breasts (typically
    180g)
juice of 1 lime
1 small cauliflower head
    (typically 200g)
½ large red onion,
    peeled and diced
1 large tomato, diced
1½ jalapeño peppers, diced
1 small or ½ large avocado,
    peeled and diced
seasoning, to taste

1 Season the chicken and leave in a bowl
to marinate with half the lime juice.

2 Break the cauliflower into florets and place
in a food processor and whizz, or grate with
a cheese grater until riced. Season to taste.

3 Place the onion, tomato and jalapeño in
a bowl and squeeze over the remaining lime.
Mix together well.

4 Preheat the grill to medium-high.

5 Place the chicken under the grill and cook
for 15–20 minutes, turning after half the time.

6 Meanwhile, warm the cauliflower in a
microwave for 1–2 minutes.

7 Remove from the microwave and stir in
the diced vegetables and their lime juice.

8 Tip the vegetables onto a serving plate,
slice the grilled chicken and place it on top.
Scatter with the diced avocado, season to
taste and serve.

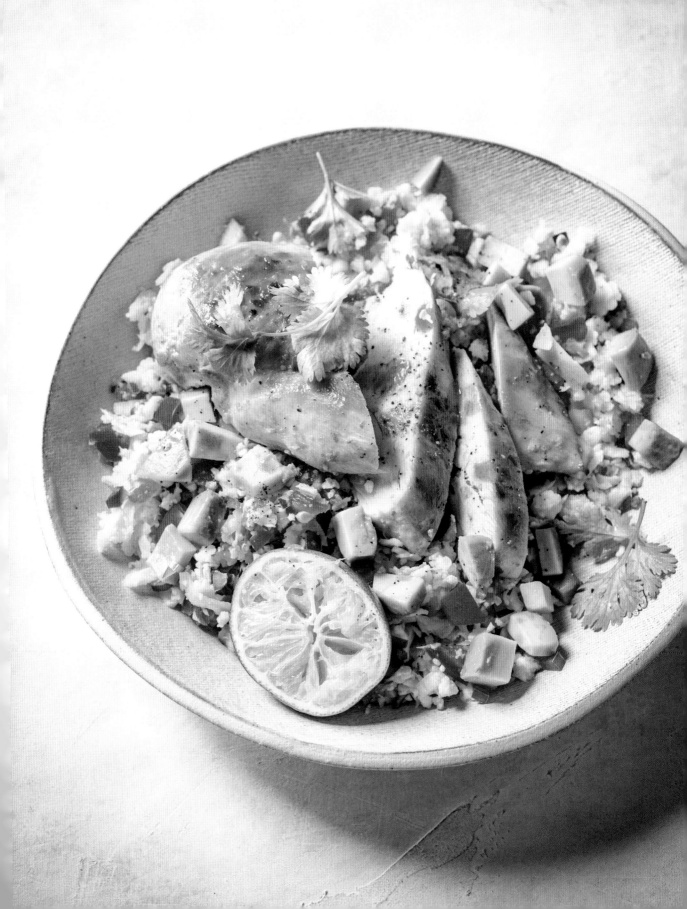

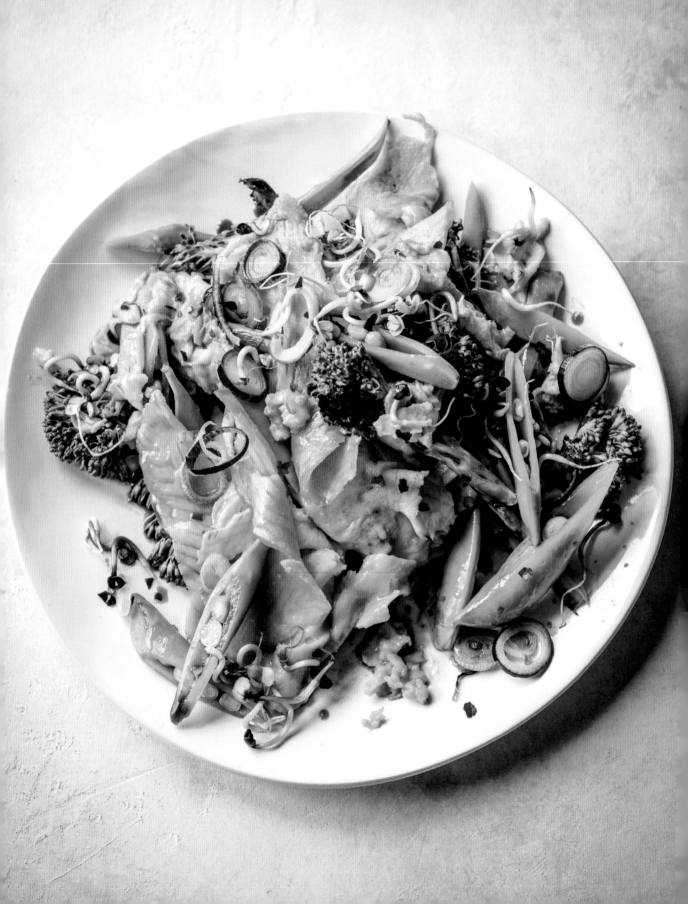

Smoked Salmon Stir-Fry

Sprinkle the veg with five-spice powder before
stir-frying, for an Asian twist.

SERVES 1

Quantities for Women

1 tbsp sesame oil

150g mixed vegetables,
 finely sliced or ½ pack
 ready-prepared stir-fry veg

2 whole eggs

2 tbsp soy sauce

100g smoked salmon, torn
 into pieces

seasoning, to taste

Quantities for Men

1½ tbsp sesame oil

225g mixed vegetables,
 finely sliced or 1 pack
 ready-prepared stir-
 fry veg

3 whole eggs

3 tbsp soy sauce

150g smoked salmon,
 torn into pieces

seasoning, to taste

1 Place the sesame oil in a frying pan over
a medium heat.

2 Add the veg to the pan and stir-fry for
3–4 minutes.

3 Depending on your preference, you can
either crack the eggs into the pan and stir-fry
everything together for 1–2 minutes, or whisk
the eggs in a bowl and cook them in separate
pan to make an omelette. In this case, slice and
stir through the cooked veg before serving.

4 Add the soy sauce to the pan and stir to coat.

5 Tip onto a plate, top with the salmon, season
to taste and serve.

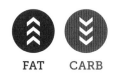

FAT   **CARB**

Hearty Salad

Salads can be even more filling than a steak, if you
do them right! I sprinkle paprika on my chicken breast
before grilling, for a little kick.

SERVES 1

Quantities for Women
1 chicken breast (typically
    120g)
1 small egg
½ iceberg lettuce,
    shredded finely
1 small tomato, diced
½ avocado, peeled and diced
1 tsp olive oil
seasoning, to taste

Quantities for Men
1½ chicken breasts
    (typically 180g)
1 large egg
¾ iceberg lettuce,
    shredded finely
1 large tomato, diced
1 small or ½ large avocado,
    peeled and diced
1½ tsp olive oil
seasoning, to taste

1 Preheat the grill to medium-high.

2 Season the chicken breast and place under
the grill. Cook for 15–20 minutes, turning after
half the time.

3 Meanwhile, bring a small pan of water to
the boil, add the egg and cook for 5–6 minutes.
Remove from the pan, leave to cool and then
peel and slice.

4 Combine the lettuce, tomato and avocado
in a serving bowl. Slice the chicken and place
on top with the sliced egg.

5 Drizzle with the olive oil, season to taste
and serve.

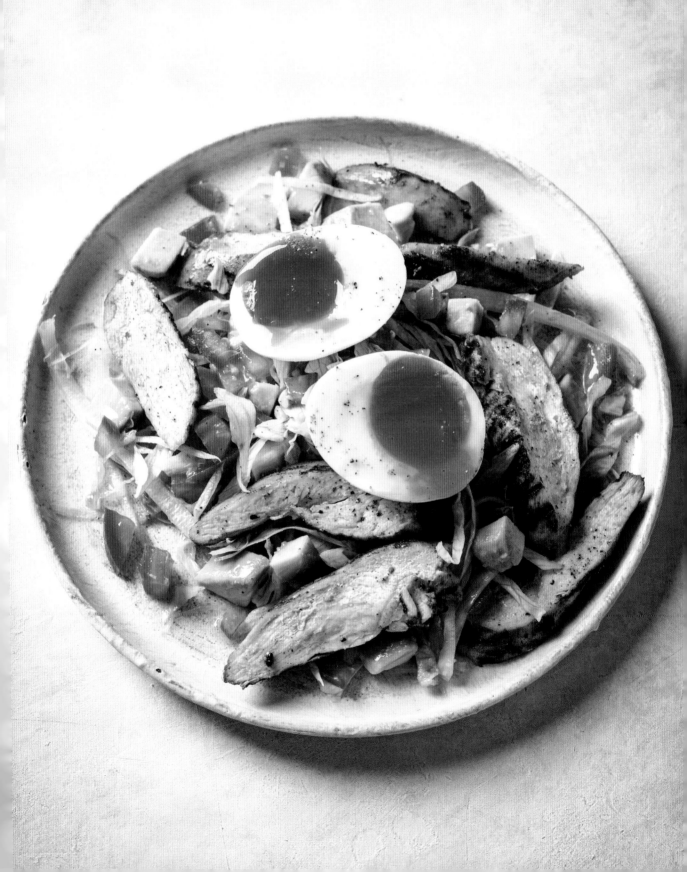

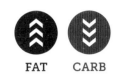

FAT   **CARB**

Hearty Soup

The nuttiness of the pine nuts goes so well with the broccoli in this soup. Adding some freshly ground black pepper and picked basil leaves would take it to another level.

SERVES 1

Quantities for Women

1 chicken breast
   (typically 120g)
1 small broccoli head, broken
   into florets (typically 200g)
1 level tbsp salted butter
2 level tbsp pine nuts
seasoning, to taste

Quantities for Men

1½ chicken breasts
   (typically 180g)
1 large broccoli head, broken
   into florets (typically 300g)
1 heaped tbsp salted butter
3 level tbsp pine nuts
seasoning, to taste

1 Preheat the grill to medium-high.

2 Season the chicken breast and cook under the grill for 15–20 minutes, turning after half the time.

3 Meanwhile, bring a large pan of salted water to the boil, add the broccoli and cook for 20 minutes (you need to cook it to within an inch of its life – the broccoli has to be very soft).

4 Drain two thirds of the water from the broccoli pan, leaving the rest in the pan.

5 Add the butter and half the pine nuts to the pan and either pour the contents into a blender or use a hand blender to whizz the soup to the desired consistency.

6 Pour back into the pan to reheat, if necessary, then check the seasoning.

7 Remove the chicken breast from the grill and shred, using two forks.

8 Stir half the chicken into the soup and pour into a serving bowl.

9 Top the soup with the remaining shredded chicken and pine nuts, season to taste and serve.

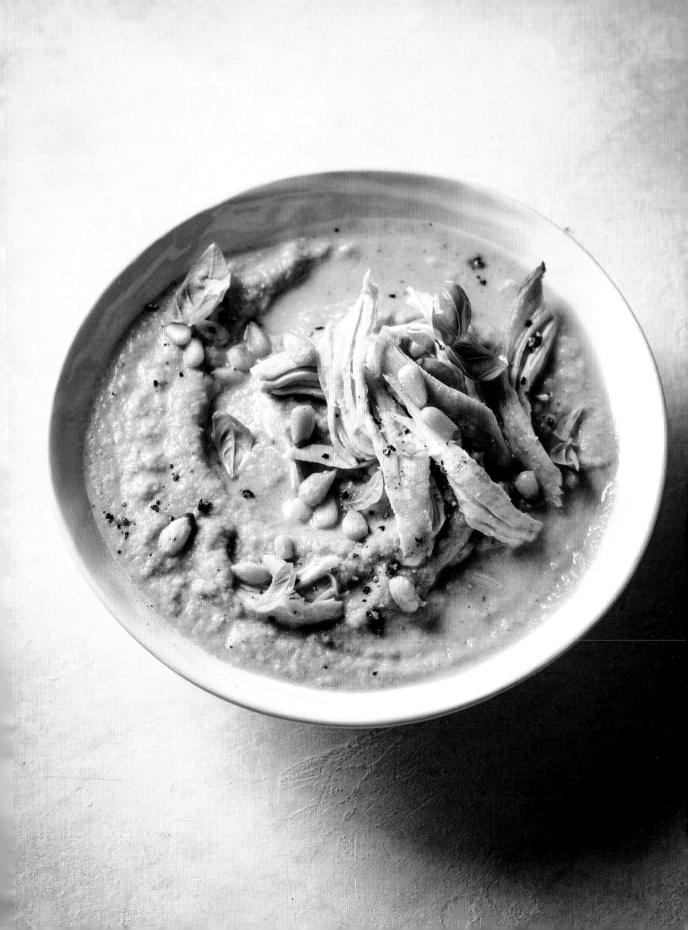

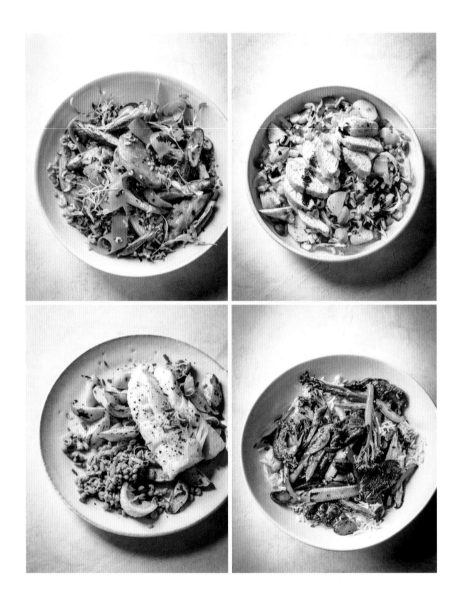

HIGH CARB
LUNCHES
AND
DINNERS
LOW FAT

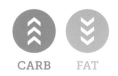

CARB **FAT**

Steak and Sweet Potato Mash

Add a clove of garlic to the sweet potato as you boil
it to give your mash some added flavour.

SERVES 1

Quantities for Women

1 small lean steak
(typically 150–200g)
1 small sweet potato
(typically 150–200g),
peeled and quartered
dash of unsweetened
almond milk
seasoning, to taste

Quantities for Men

1 large lean steak (typically
225–300g)
1 large sweet potato
(typically 225–300g),
peeled and quartered
dash of unsweetened
almond milk
seasoning, to taste

1 Allow the steak to sit and come up to
room temperature before cooking.

2 Bring a large pan of salted water to the
boil, add the sweet potato and cook for
20–30 minutes.

3 Drain the potato, return to the pan and
add the almond milk. Season well and mash.
Keep warm until ready to serve.

4 Place a frying pan over a high heat and
leave it to become smoking hot.

5 Season the steak, then sear in the pan on
each side for 1 minute, or until cooked to
your preference.

6 Remove the steak from the pan, check the
seasoning and serve alongside the sweet
potato mash.

CARB   FAT

Chicken Sausage and Chips

I like to sprinkle paprika over the wedges before roasting them in the oven.

SERVES 1

Quantities for Women

1 small sweet potato (typically 150–200g), washed and cut into wedges

4 chicken sausages

seasoning, to taste

Quantities for Men

1 large sweet potato (typically 225–300g), washed and cut into wedges

6 chicken sausages

seasoning, to taste

1 Preheat the oven to 200°C and line a roasting tin with baking parchment.

2 Season the potato wedges then place in the prepared tin and cook in the oven for 20–30 minutes.

3 Meanwhile, preheat the grill to medium-high.

4 Pierce the chicken sausages with a fork and cook under the grill for 15 minutes, turning occasionally.

5 Check the wedges for seasoning and then serve them with the sausages.

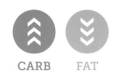

CARB FAT

Chicken Stir-Fry

Add Chinese five-spice powder or ground coriander
to the veg or chicken before you stir-fry, or liven things
up by garnishing the finished dish with fresh herbs
– try fresh coriander or parsley.

SERVES 1

Quantities for Women

1 chicken breast (typically
   120g), sliced thickly
2 tbsp soy sauce
150g mixed vegetables
   (such as courgette, carrot
   and baby corn), sliced
   finely or ½ pack ready-
   prepared stir-fry veg
½ microwaveable pack any
   rice (typically 125g)
seasoning, to taste

Quantities for Men

1½ chicken breasts (typically
   180g), sliced thickly
3 tbsp soy sauce
225g mixed vegetables
   (such as courgette, carrot
   and baby corn), sliced
   finely or 1 pack ready-
   prepared stir-fry veg
1 microwaveable pack of
   any rice (typically 250g)
seasoning, to taste

1 Place the chicken in a bowl and mix with
the soy sauce.

2 Place a non-stick pan over a medium
heat, add the chicken and soy and stir-fry
for 4–5 minutes, or until lightly browned.

3 Add the veg to the pan and stir-fry for
3–4 minutes to soften.

4 Add the rice and stir-fry for a further
2–3 minutes.

5 Tip into a bowl, check the seasoning
and serve.

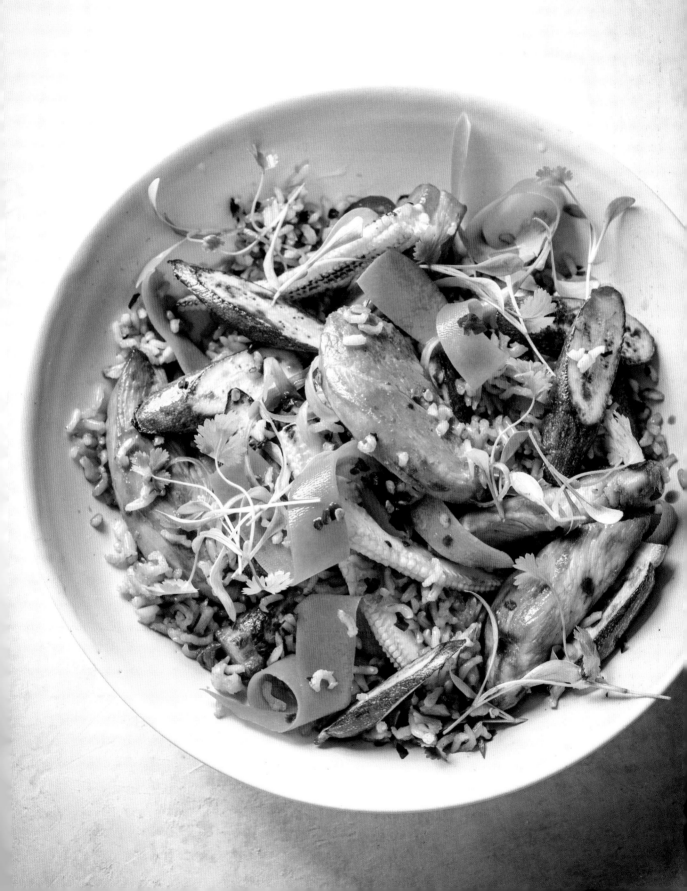

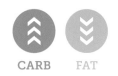

Mexican Rice Bowl

I like to add a dash of Tabasco and a pinch of chilli powder
or paprika to the chicken before cooking.

SERVES 1

Quantities for Women
1 chicken breast
    (typically 120g)
juice of ½ lime
½ microwaveable pack of
    any rice (typically 125g)
½ small red onion, diced
1 small tomato, diced
1 jalapeño pepper, diced
seasoning, to taste

Quantities for Men
1½ chicken breasts
    (typically 180g)
juice of 1 lime
1 microwaveable pack of
    any rice (typically 250g)
½ large red onion, diced
1 large tomato, diced
1½ jalapeño peppers, diced
seasoning, to taste

1 Place the chicken in a bowl with half the
lime juice.

2 Preheat the grill to medium-high.

3 Place the chicken under the grill and cook
for 15–20 minutes, turning after half the time.

4 Heat the rice in the microwave according to
the packet instructions (typically 2 minutes).

5 Tip the rice into a bowl and add the red onion,
tomato and jalapeño.

6 Pour over the remaining lime juice and
mix again.

7 Place the grilled chicken on top of the rice
and veg, check the seasoning and serve.

Chicken and Rice

This takes a bit longer to make than some of the other recipes in this book but it's a great one to double up the quantities on so you have a meal already prepared for another day.

SERVES 1

Quantities for Women

½ onion, peeled and diced
1 tsp chopped garlic
1 large handful button
   mushrooms, diced
1 small celery stalk, diced
½ small red pepper, diced
½ small green pepper, diced
1 chicken breast (typically
   120g), cubed or diced
1 chicken stock cube
½ microwaveable pack of
   any rice (typically 125g)
seasoning, to taste

Quantities for Men

½ onion, peeled and diced
1½ tsp chopped garlic
1½ large handfuls button
   mushrooms, diced
1 large celery stalk, diced
½ large red pepper, diced
½ large green pepper, diced
1½ chicken breasts (typically
   180g), cubed or diced
1 chicken stock cube
1 microwaveable pack of
   any rice (typically 250g)
seasoning, to taste

1 Place a large non-stick pan over a medium heat and add the onion, garlic, mushrooms, celery and both peppers. Fry for 4–5 minutes, or until soft. Season to taste.

2 Add the chicken to the pan, stir and fry for 4–5 minutes, or until lightly browned. Check the seasoning.

3 Dissolve the stock cube in 300ml boiling water and pour this into the pan with the chicken and vegetables. Leave to simmer for 30–40 minutes.

4 Heat the rice in the microwave according to the packet instructions (typically 2 minutes) and tip into a serving bowl.

5 Pour the chicken stew over the rice, check the seasoning and serve.

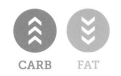

CARB   FAT

Warm Chicken Potato Salad

Fresh herbs like parsley and basil will add another dimension to this salad.

SERVES 1

Quantities for Women
2 tbsp balsamic vinegar
1 chicken breast
    (typically 120g)
5 small new potatoes
½ iceberg lettuce,
    shredded finely
1 small tomato, diced
½ cucumber, diced
½ small red onion,
    peeled and diced
2 level tbsp tinned sweetcorn
seasoning, to taste

Quantities for Men
3 tbsp balsamic vinegar
1½ chicken breasts
    (typically 180g)
8 small new potatoes
1 iceberg lettuce,
    shredded finely
1 large tomato, diced
¾ cucumber, diced
½ large red onion,
    peeled and diced
3 level tbsp tinned sweetcorn
seasoning, to taste

1 Preheat the grill to medium-high.

2 Drizzle half the balsamic vinegar over the chicken breast and cook under the grill for 15–20 minutes, turning after half the time.

3 Meanwhile, bring a pan of salted water to the boil, add the new potatoes and cook for 10–15 minutes. Drain and cut into halves or quarters.

4 Place the lettuce, tomato, cucumber and red onion in a bowl and mix together well.

5 Top with the potato and sprinkle with the sweetcorn.

6 Remove the chicken from the grill and slice before placing on top of the salad.

7 Drizzle with the remaining balsamic vinegar, season to taste and serve.

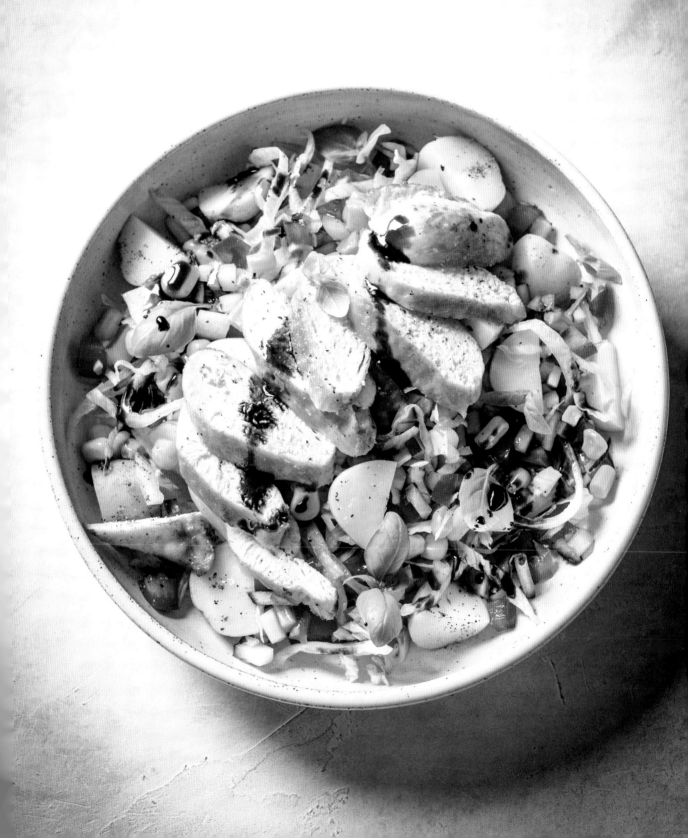

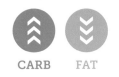

CARB   FAT

Fish, Chips and Mushy Peas

Splash vinegar on your chips, if that's how you like them,
and sprinkle the fish with snipped chives and lemon zest.

SERVES 1

Quantities for Women
10 small new potatoes,
   quartered
1 large fillet any white fish
   (typically 150g)
juice of ½ lemon
1 large handful frozen peas
dash of unsweetened
   almond milk
seasoning, to taste

Quantities for Men
15 small new potatoes,
   quartered
1½ large fillets any white fish
   (typically 225g)
juice of 1 lemon
1½ large handfuls
   frozen peas
dash of unsweetened
   almond milk
seasoning, to taste

1 Preheat the oven to 220°C.

2 Bring a pan of salted water to the boil, add
the potatoes and cook for 10–15 minutes.

3 Drain the potatoes and lay them out on
a large baking tray.

4 Season the fish with salt, pepper and the
lemon juice and place on the tray beside the
potatoes. Season and cook in the oven for
10–15 minutes.

5 Meanwhile, bring a small pan of water to the
boil and cook the peas for 3–4 minutes. Drain
and return to the pan with the almond milk.
Season to taste and mash with a fork.

6 Remove the fish and chips from the oven
and serve alongside the mushy peas.

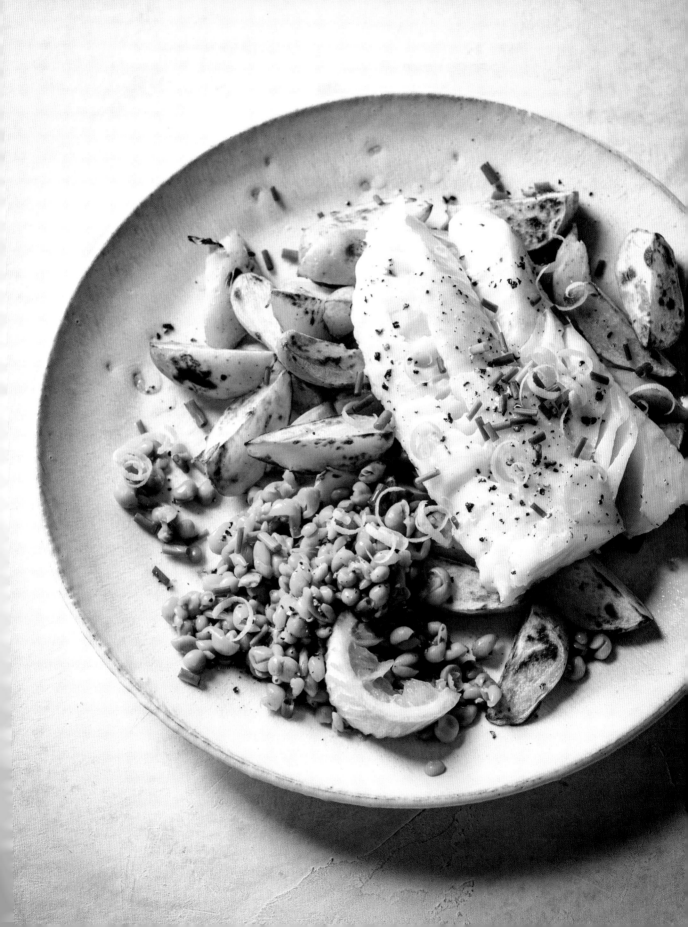

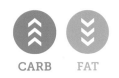

CARB FAT

Fish Pie

A delicious alternative to a traditional fish pie.

SERVES 1

Quantities for Women

1 small baking potato,
    peeled and quartered
dash of unsweetened
    almond milk
1 leek, sliced into 2cm circles
3 level tbsp 0% fat Greek
    yoghurt
3 level tbsp frozen peas
1 small fillet any white fish
    (typically 100g)
juice of ½ lemon
1 handful prawns
seasoning, to taste

Quantities for Men

1 large baking potato,
    peeled and quartered
dash of unsweetened
    almond milk
1½ leeks, sliced into
    2cm circles
4 heaped tbsp 0% fat
    Greek yoghurt
4 heaped tbsp frozen peas
1 large fillet any white fish
    (typically 150g)
juice of 1 lemon
1½ handfuls prawns
seasoning, to taste

1 Preheat the oven to 200°C.

2 Bring a pan of salted water to the boil, add the potato and cook for 15–20 minutes. Drain and return to the pan, add the almond milk, season to taste and mash.

3 Place the leek in the bottom of a small baking dish (roughly 20cm) and season.

4 Spread a third of the Greek yoghurt over the leeks and top with a third of the peas.

5 Lay the fish on top of the peas and season with salt, pepper and half the lemon juice.

6 Spread half the remaining Greek yoghurt over the fish and top with half the remaining peas.

7 Lay the prawns on top of the peas and season with salt, pepper and the remaining lemon juice.

8 Smear the remaining Greek yoghurt over the prawns and top with the remaining peas.

9 Cover with the mash and bake in the oven for 20–25 minutes, or until bubbling at the sides and browning on top.

CARB FAT

Sunday Roast

The gravy completes the dish perfectly!

SERVES 1

Quantities for Women

1 small baking potato,
    peeled and quartered
1 chicken sausage
1 chicken breast
    (typically 120g)
1 large handful frozen peas
1 large handful broccoli
    florets
1 tbsp gravy granules
seasoning, to taste

Quantities for Men

1 large baking potato,
    peeled and quartered
1½ chicken sausages
1 large chicken breast
    (typically 180g)
1½ large handfuls
    frozen peas
1½ large handfuls
    broccoli florets
1 tbsp gravy granules
seasoning, to taste

1 Preheat the oven to 200°C.

2 Bring a pan of salted water to the boil,
add the potato and cook for 15–20 minutes.

3 Drain the potato and place on a baking tray.
Leave to cool slightly before smushing with
the heel of your hand and seasoning. Add
the sausage to the tray and cook both in
the oven for 10 minutes.

4 Remove the tray from the oven and add
the chicken breast, alongside the sausage
and potato. Season it well and return the tray
to the oven for a further 10–15 minutes,
or until cooked through.

5 Meanwhile, bring a pan of salted water to
the boil, add the peas and broccoli and cook
for 4–5 minutes. Drain and return to the pan
and keep warm until ready to serve.

6 Mix the gravy granules with 200ml boiling
water from the kettle in a small jug.

7 Remove the potatoes, chicken sausage
and chicken breast from the oven and serve
alongside the peas, broccoli and gravy.

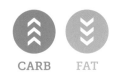

CARB FAT

Chilli Beef and Rice

You can add paprika and ground cumin to the marinade,
if you like it spicy.

SERVES 1

Quantities for Women

1 small lean steak (typically
  150–200g), sliced thinly
2 tbsp soy sauce
2 tbsp hot sauce
1 tsp chopped garlic
1 chilli, chopped finely
150g mixed vegetables,
  sliced finely or ½ pack
  ready-prepared stir-fry veg
½ microwaveable pack of
  any rice (typically 125g)
seasoning, to taste

Quantities for Men

1 large lean steak (typically
  225–300g), sliced thinly
3 tbsp soy sauce
3 tbsp hot sauce
1½ tsp chopped garlic
1½ chillies, chopped finely
225g mixed vegetables,
  sliced finely or 1 pack
  ready-prepared stir-fry veg
1 microwaveable pack of any
  rice (typically 250g)
seasoning, to taste

1 Place the steak in a bowl and cover with half
the soy sauce, half the hot sauce, half the garlic
and half the chilli.

2 Place a non-stick pan over a high heat and
leave it to become smoking hot.

3 Add the beef and its marinade and cook for
1–2 minutes.

4 Add the veg and the remaining soy sauce,
hot sauce, garlic and chilli, and cook for a
further 3–4 minutes.

5 Meanwhile, heat the rice in the microwave
according to the packet instructions, then tip
into a bowl.

6 Check the seasoning then serve the chilli
beef with the rice.

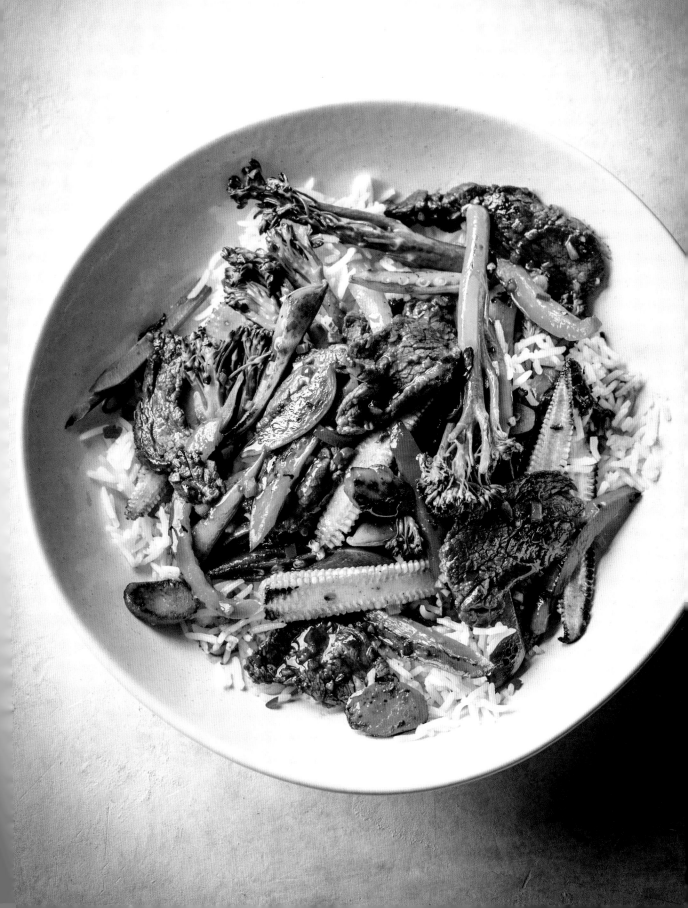

TRACKING YOUR PROGRESS

As a Personal Trainer, I don't always recommend tracking your progress. Weighing scales, progress pictures, measurements, body fat callipers – these methods only come into their own when a client is 100% serious about their body transformation.

When I know that a client is genuinely serious, that's when I'll ask for weekly or fortnightly check-ins. That way, I can see if I need to make any changes to their diet or training as the weeks roll on.

Hopefully, you've bought this book because you, too, are serious about your body transformation, so if you want to track your progress, here's how to do it.

WEIGHING SCALES

First and foremost, you should understand that there are a number of different factors that affect your weight on the scales, which is why they can be so misleading when it comes to results. Water retention, in particular, wreaks havoc at weigh-ins and can be caused by:

» Cortisol (stress) levels – both physical (training) and mental (work)
» Daily / weekly sodium intake
» Daily / weekly fibre intake
» Daily / weekly water intake
» Daily / weekly carbohydrate intake
» Muscle gain / loss
» Fat gain / loss
» Menstrual cycle
» Alcohol
» The list goes on (and on)...

However, scales can be a good way to measure progress, for beginners in particular. If you choose to weigh in, I want you to use the following method.

Make sure you weigh yourself first thing in the morning with no food or drink in your system. Make a note of your weight on the following days:

» Day 1, Week 1
» Day 1, Week 2
» Day 1, Week 3
» Day 1, Week 4

Don't forget, though, that the results can be misleading. If you weigh in after a high carb day, for example, the scales will absolutely jump. And if they do jump up, it's most likely because glycogen acts like a sponge and pulls water into the muscle. If they jump down, however, it's most likely because of something we call the 'whoosh' effect – when your body drops a lot of weight quickly after being re-fed. Plus, if you're coming up to or are on your menstrual cycle, I honestly wouldn't even bother with the scales.

PROGRESS PICTURES

Progress pictures are a great way to see changes that you probably won't notice on a day-to-day basis. However, you should only take pics once a fortnight at the most, as aesthetic changes take time.

If you do choose to take progress pictures, I want you to use the following method.

Make sure you take them first thing in the morning with no food or drink in your system. Stand in front of a mirror and take a photo front on and side on, on the following days:

>> Day 1, Week 1

>> Day 1, Week 3

>> Day 7, Week 4

Compare your week 1 side on photo and your week 4 side on photo and, if you have stayed 100% on track with your diet and training, you'll be astounded!

MEASUREMENTS

It's a great idea to log your measurements on a fortnightly basis. If you choose to track using measurements, I want you to use the following method.

First thing in the morning with no food or drink in your system and using a flexible tape measure (the material kind is best):

>> Measure your upper arm (around the bicep)

>> Measure your chest circumference (widest girth of back and chest)

>> Measure your waist circumference (narrowest girth)

>> Measure your upper leg (widest girth of upper thigh)

Take these measurements on:

>> Day 1, Week 1

>> Day 1, Week 3

>> Day 7, Week 4

BODY FAT % – CALLIPERS

Let me start by saying that I do not endorse body fat measurements by machine – I've been told I have 13% body fat many times and have had various machines tell me I'm 23% or more. Measuring body fat with callipers (or booking a DEXA scan, but that can be expensive) is the most accurate way to track aesthetic progress.

Callipers look like little pincers and you pinch areas of your skin (lower stomach, inner thigh, etc) to calculate your overall Body Fat %.

You can either order callipers online and read the instructions on how to measure your BF% or, if you are a member of a gym, ask a Personal Trainer if he / she can show you how to do it.

I recommend doing this no more than once a fortnight, though. Don't be disheartened if you only see a tiny drop – anything over 1% is a success. If your BF has decreased by any decimals whatsoever, you are on the right track!

WHAT NEXT?

As I write this, I am hopeful that
the majority of you have now completed
The 4-Week Body Blitz.

If you've been circuit training 5–6 days per week,
sticking 100% to the calorie-controlled, carb-cycled diet
(no cheating!) then you should have seen results from
weeks 1–2 all the way into week 4.

However, it's not always this linear. We cannot tell our
bodies when to change and by how much – if we could
we'd all be in perfect shape all the time.

The fact is that for most of us, some weeks nothing
happens at all and other weeks you can see a big drop
on the scales or in the mirror. This is totally normal
and it's important to remember that, as long as you
are training hard and following your diet to the letter,
the results WILL COME.

If you're now at a loss as to what to do next in terms of
your diet and training, I suggest you continue with this
plan for up to 12 weeks in total. The calories are low but
maintainable and the high carb days are frequent enough
to see you comfortably through each week of training.

If you find that after a few weeks you plateau, add another
5 minutes onto your circuits. It has taken me a long time

to get there, but I can now circuit train at a high intensity for up to an hour. I'd recommend one hour as the cut off point for circuit training specifically, but there's no reason why you can't take up another form of exercise, such as weight lifting, a gym class or a new sport.

No matter what you choose to do, I suggest training for a minimum of 5 days a week and dietary 'cheating' for no more than 1 night a week (instead of a high carb day) if you want to achieve and / or maintain results.

If you weren't able to complete the 4 weeks giving 100% to the training, diet or both, don't panic, you can try again.

Remember – it takes time to implement changes and forge new habits, and sometimes you need to have an epic fail before you can achieve epic success. This book was designed to get you moving and eating for aesthetic results in a 4-week time period, but training and nutrition goes far beyond *The 4-Week Body Blitz*.

Have a look at my website, FitnessFondue.com, and my social media pages, @madeleychloe on Instagram and Twitter, to get more information on how I get myself and my clients into great shape.

In the end, if I'm honest, it's no longer about how I look for me. I simply feel better knowing I'm fit and healthy – especially when that well-earned cheat day rolls around!

INDEX

ACKNOWLEDGEMENTS

First and foremost, thank you to my friends and family for having faith that my constant gym selfies were part of a bigger picture! I know you all hated seeing my half-naked body online every day, but I told you people would get it eventually!

Next, to my wonderful partner, James Haskell, who was incensed that I didn't have a book deal and insisted I meet with his agent. We've been through a hell of a lot, kiddo, but your tenacity was the missing link in my life, and I am so lucky to call you my partner in crime.

To my agent, Clare Hulton, who believed in me from day one and pushed everyone else to believe in me, too. Thank you.

To my editor, Michelle Signore, who lets me be my crazy self and never bats an eyelid!

To my marketing guru, Emma Burton, for sharing my OCD tendencies and love of Disney. Your communication skills are second to none, which I suppose is why you're so good at your job!

To Becky Short, *The 4-Week Body Blitz* publicist! You kept me in the loop from day 1 and always came up with such fun ideas! I am beyond lucky to have you helping me spread the word!

To Jo Roberts-Miller, who put up with my militant, panicked ramblings and edited my book in a way that made me feel 100% comfortable and excited.

To the wonderful Sam Riley, who took the images for this book and never fails to impress me with his work ethic, positive attitude and sheer skill. You and Leo made those gruelling shooting days so much fun for me, and I adore the pants off you both!

To Smith and Gilmour for making this book look so beautiful! It is prettier than I ever could have imagined! THANK YOU for all your hard work!

And lastly, to my fitness following, especially those of you who've been in my corner since day one. It's a weird thing, getting to know people over social media. I am a cynic who scoffs at online 'friendships'. However, my online relationships with all of you have felt very real to me and have seen me through many dark days. I hope I have returned the favour and it goes without saying that this book is for you. I hope it answers your questions about how I do things. I hope it gets you the results you deserve. Thank you, from the bottom of my heart, for your continued love and support.

xxx